Colour Scents

SUZY CHIAZZARI

Colour Scents

Healing with Colour and Aroma

INDEX COMPILED BY MARY KIRKNESS

ILLUSTRATIONS BY THE AUTHOR

SAFFRON WALDEN
THE C.W. DANIEL COMPANY LIMITED

First published in Great Britain in 1998
by The C.W. Daniel Company Limited
1 Church Path, Saffron Walden,
Essex, CB10 1JP, United Kingdom

© Suzy Chiazzari 1998

ISBN 0 85207 316 X

Produced by
Book Production Consultants plc,
25–27 High Street, Chesterton, Cambridge CB4 1ND
Typeset by Cambridge Photosetting Services
Printed and bound by Hillman Printers (Frome), Limited, England.

Contents

*This book is dedicated to my mother who nurtured my creativity
and my father whose love of nature has always been an inspiration to me.
I also wish to thank all the colour therapists and aromatherapists
who have lovingly shared their knowledge
and given me encouragement with this venture.*

Foreword

by Patricia Davis

There are many ways of understanding essential oils and each of them offers us a different perspective – opens a different door, if you like.

We may look at the unique biochemistry of a plant, or at the way it affects our emotions; its colour, shape and habit of growth, or the specific bacteria it will counteract. We may consider an essential oil from a purely physical point of view – as a beauty-aid or to relieve aching muscles – or we may value it for its subtle, spiritual qualities. The beauty and wonder of essential oils is that they are all of these things. So many books on the subject, though, deal only with the physical nature of the oils.

Suzy Chiazzari's book comes as a breath of fresh ... and very fragrant ... air, for its opens up a new perspective on the role of aromatherapy in vibrational medicine by allying it intimately with the sister-discipline of colour healing. Being myself a painter as well as an aromatherapist, I have long been fascinated by the parallels between colours and aromas but nowhere have I seen these parallels explored as excitingly and with such sensitivity as in this book.

The fact that aromatics can heal is well established: that colours can do so to is equally true, even if not so widely acknowledged. Bringing the two together as Suzy does adds a new dimension, a synthesis of healing powers that is as exciting as it is profound.

Here is a book with something new and original to say. I hope you enjoy it as much as I have.

Preface

One only has to look into the centre of a newly opened rose to be transported, for a moment, into a mystical place beyond space and time. Our physical senses of sight and smell are the doors to our individual time capsule and once through them we can experience the world in a new and wonderful way. Through the beauty of nature we are transported out of our ego-centred world into one which connects us with other dimensions and the great cosmic forces. In this multi-dimensional place we can discover who we really are, so that our body, mind and spirit become integrated and we can be at one with ourselves. In this place we know we are 'embodied' spirits and we can meet with beings from other realms, the devas of the plants and trees, angelic helpers and the great beings of light who are the ascended spiritual masters.

Unfortunately, we are only able to hold on to this mystical moment every now and again, and once we have been through the door our soul craves to return to this wonderful place which is its true home. Our life would be a very sad one if we were to spend it continuously wanting to escape from this physical world, but through the love of mother earth, we have been given the gifts of colour and aroma to use during our time on this planet for restoring wholeness to the different parts of our being. If we take care of these gifts and use them wisely we will find fulfilment, peace and contentment for the purity of the vibrations bring harmony to our mind, body and spirit and can actively keep us in good health.

Colour Scents grew out of the desire to show the world that we all have access to the secrets of these two mystical forces and that our awareness can be heightened at any stage in our lives. I was most fortunate to become aware of the power and beauty of colour and aroma at an early age.

As a small child I was always drawn to the beautiful colours and shapes of flowers, plants and trees in the tropical city of Durban, South Africa. Here the profusion of lush foliage, brightly coloured and heavily scented flowers surrounded me. It was a place where all the senses were stimulated. Overhead was the deep blue sky and golden sun, and around me the swaying palm fronds, crimson hibiscus and sweet smelling Frangipani and there was the ever-changing sea. I started drawing and painting my world and found that the colours and scents I wanted to portray became interchangeable. The scents carried on the wind would conjure up images of moving colours and the colours themselves provoked wonderful perfumes. The experience was intensely personal and one which has brought me a sense of well-being and joy throughout my life.

My holidays were spent on a farm playing under tall oaks, cypress and pines, many of which were planted by my grandmother thirty years before. The long hours I spent alone allowed me to live in a special world where my friends were the animals, birds, trees and flowers. My Irish Grandmother had told me about fairy rings and I found secret places around the garden and hills which were inhabited by spirits, fairies and elves.

As I played I was also intensely aware of invisible friends watching over me, and the angels became my guardians through the long months when my mother went away to America. Over the years, I have come to know my guardian angels well and they have sustained me through many hard times. They have also revealed to me many things about my life and this world, and it is through their guidance that I later came to understand the real extent of the gifts of colour and aroma.

Although I had worked in the field of art and design since leaving college, I knew from personal experience that colour was more than a tool for creating a pleasing environment and that it embodied life-giving and nurturing properties. It became my quest to find out more about this force which through its own transmutation could travel so easily between our visible and the invisible worlds. My studies took me on another journey, where I met many wonderful people who wished to share their knowledge and experiences of the mysteries of life. It was through the unfolding of the petals of life that I met my teacher Marie Louise Lacy, who initiated me into the therapeutic and esoteric aspects of healing with colour. It all made perfect sense to me, and I understood that we have the ability to access knowledge through our higher mind and that our angelic guardians are always there to assist us, when we humbly ask for help. Marie Louise also reinforced the idea that aroma and colour were inextricably linked, and since then I have had the honour to work with several aromatherapists in understanding the links between these two powerful but subtle forces.

I share with you in this book the discoveries made through these many sources. They are by no means complete or definitive, and there is much work still to be done. The investigation of the relationship between colour and aroma was made with no expectations as it was important to avoid the all-time pitfall many researchers fall into, of making the findings fit the theory. It was extremely exciting and rewarding when the healing qualities, revealed through the colour signatures of essential oils, correlated so closely with the therapeutic uses of the oils in Aromatherapy. Hopefully, through this means, we can increase our understanding about their effects of colour and aroma on our subtle bodies.

In *Colour Scents* I have tried to create a framework which will help you make sense of your own experiences of colour and aroma and hopefully, like me, you will also be inspired to forge the links between these special divine gifts and use them with reverence for personal growth and healing.

The information given in this book is not intended to replace orthodox medical treatment. Although most of the suggestions allow you to use colour and aroma oneself for healing, certain light instruments and essential oils should only be administered under the guidance of a qualified practitioner.

Introduction

OUR LOST SIXTH SENSE

When humankind lived in harmony with nature, we revered the power of the sun and honoured the earth. We made use of the basic elements of sunlight and magnetic earth energy for healing and to reinforce our cosmic connections. The use of colourful and aromatic healing plants and herbs formed a major part of nearly all ancient cultures, especially in their religious ceremonies and spiritual practices. The burning and smoking of aromatic resins, herbs and spices was an integral part of these ceremonies with colour being used as inspiration and focus for meditation. The light reflective qualities and healing properties of rocks and gemstones were also used to attract prosperity, longevity and health.

Colours have always had symbolic significance, the robes worn by priests and healers and those adorning the places of worship were carefully chosen for the qualities they represented. In many ancient civilisations, colours were related to the planets and elemental forces and offerings of scented flowers reflecting these colours were made to gods and deities.

The view of the universe and everything as a moving mass of connected and interdependent energy allowed the ancients to accept the connections between many healing forces both seen and unseen. Our perception of time was not so delineated as it is today and it was recognised that it is the constantly changing energy and its transformation that denotes time. For many centuries, it was accepted that ancestral spirits and those of the newly deceased were ever present and interacted with our physical dimension. Some groups, like the aboriginal people of Australia, still recognise the existence of 'dreamtime' which extends outside space and time, and many Eastern cultures believe that we exist on a multi-dimensional level during our life on earth.

The belief in mutual exchange of energy in all life, allows us to accept the connections between the vibrational forces of light, sound and aroma. When we were more sensitive to other dimensions our conscious mind did not form a barrier between our analytical and intuitive side allowing us to experience the world in a more complete and holistic way. In times when our sensory perception was highly developed, we were also sensitive to vibrations relating to emotions and mind waves.

The ability to perceive vibrations of all kinds is not peculiar to the human race as many other animals experience the world through heightened sensory perception. There are hundreds of known cases of animals being aware of events and intentions of people well out of their sensory range. Extra-sensory perception provides access to areas outside our every day human experience and in the days when we lived in harmony with nature we too had a strongly developed sixth sense. The more we moved away from our connection with the natural world, the more specialised and restricted our sensory perception has become and as the emphasis on the physical world increases, the less able we are to perceive and enter the spiritual planes and experience the world on a multi-dimensional level.

While sight has become our dominant sense, our memory of odour is much more long-lasting than our visual memory. Some of our oldest memories are connected with scent. Often we can remember the smell of our family home, school, or place we went on holiday as a very young child. For me, a whiff of lavender reminds me of my grandmother and pine needles awakens memories of my school playground.

Memory of aroma can sometimes be so great it can permeate space and time and pass with us from life time to another. The scent of orange blossom and jasmine flowers have a particularly strong association with certain places especially in the warm countries where they grow in pro-fusion. It is not unusual to find people who have strong feelings towards these aromas which they cannot explain. Smell is related to the most antique and reptilian parts of the brain which is also closely linked with the process of hunger and sexual behaviour. Our sense of smell is the first sense to develop in the foetus, giving it a unique place in its primary connection with the soul when it first enters the body of the unborn infant.

It is not so surprising, therefore, that our memory of scent could span from one life to the next. Sometimes during a relaxation or therapy session, memories from very early childhood and even our past lives can make an appearance and these can be stimulated by both colour and aroma.

Not only can we associate colour and aroma with physical places, they are very much an integral part of our own energetic make-up. Light and aroma in our aura reveals our state of evolution at soul level so that our state of body, mind and spirit is revealed by the colours and aroma permeating our aura.

It has been said of many great Saints and Spiritual Masters that they give off a beautiful light and perfume which spreads out around them and lingers long after they are gone. Jesus Christ is associated with golden light as revealed in many beautiful paintings of antiquity. St. Germain is linked to the Violet ray, the colour of pure service while St Francis is sur-rounded by the colour green showing his affinity with the natural world. These lines from a Buddhist text describe the beauty and fragrance of the radiant aura surrounding the Buddha which was reported to have extended for several miles.

Lo, like a fragrant lotus at dawn of day with full blown virgin scent,
Behold the Buddha's glory shining forth,
As in the vaulted heaven beams the sun.

We too have our own colours and aroma which pervade our aura and reflect the energy in our physical, mental and emotional bodies. These energy vibrations spread out around us like ripples in a pond and interact with other vibrations in the environment. When we pass near someone, there is an interchange of energy and most of us have experienced good or bad vibrations coming from other people.

The fine vibrations of light and aroma also permeate solid matter and become embedded into the walls, furniture and furnishings. Often we can walk into a room and the atmosphere there will give us a strong sense of the previous occupants especially if strong emotions have been expressed in the space. Sometimes certain conditions allow these vibrations to be released and these are the times when we may see apparitions. Many old buildings which are reputed to house ghosts also have very distinctive aromas in certain rooms. Happy and loving vibrations will give a room a fresh floral scent while those places where evil deeds have occurred will result in a heavy putrid smell. People who have attended or performed exorcisms have reported the strength and affect these aromas had on them. It is through the use of powerful vibrations of light and aroma that these bad vibrations can be dissolved.

For many thousands of years our view of disease and healing was also very different from the one most people hold today. The causes of illness were seen to be much more wide-ranging and included attack from harmful energetic forces both seen and unseen. Illness affected the whole person, at many different levels, and in order to drive out the offending vibrations, the spirit as well as the body had to be cleansed and purified. Priests, spiritual healers, shamans, witch-doctors and herbalists had as important part to play in healing as medical practitioners.

Over the centuries we moved indoors away from sunlight and as modern agricultural methods took over, we have progressively lost touch with nature – the sun, the moon and the earth. As we became more manipulative and dominant of our planet, linear time has became more important to us than natural rhythms and rather than understanding the powerful healing forces around us, we have tried to create our own.

The more complex and stressful our world has become, the more our senses have become differentiated so that our brain can process and make sense of the volume of information it receives. The separation of our senses which is reflected outside and inside our own bodies is also reflected in our attitude to healing.

It was not so long ago that Hipprocrates, the father of Western medicine, practised 'holistic' medicine treating his patients with sound, colour and music as well as mineral and herbal remedies. Unfortunately, his successors ignored his use of the more subtle forms of healing, choosing to develop the more intrusive practises which have developed into the type of medicine practised to-day.

Modern medicine views our body as a number of individual parts and our healing methods are based primarily on invasive surgery and chemical interference. This reductionist approach to medicine views illness as a malfunction of its parts, and the various mechanisms of the body are understood at biological and molecular levels. The healing power of colour and aroma has also been subjected to this scientific analysis.

Aroma molecules have been shown to enter our system and the chemical messages they contain, instigating certain conscious and unconscious reactions in our system. This interpretation gives us only half the picture, for aroma also exists as vibrations which fit into the electro-magnetic spectrum normally associated with colour.

As young children we still have a strong connection to the spiritual realms and have the ability to experience the world holistically. Infants do not differentiate between the messages coming from the different sense organs and so a baby will examine an object by touch, smell, taste, as well as vision. As we grow, we learn to interpret and select sensory messages so that we perceive the world as differentiated and having orderly fashion. This need for selection, drawn from our sensory experience, is probably necessary for us to live in a modern world of such complexity. There are, however, many people who retain their childhood capacity whereby the organs of sight, smell, taste and touch are inter-connected. This ability is known as Synaesthesia, but it is usually viewed as a handicap, rather than an asset.

In most of us, the vibrations we receive through our sense of sight, hearing and smell are still so closely linked that we often associate sounds with certain colours, while colour invokes certain scents. We also associate aroma with visual colour, preferring scents of clear brightly coloured flowers, fruits and spices which conjure up the atmosphere of gardens, woodlands and citrus groves. We generally do not like the aroma of things which have dark or muddy colours such as lard, rubber, olive oil, fish, vinegar or onion and when presented with something of a dull or dark colouring our expectation is that it will have a nasty smell.

We do, therefore, still retain the ability to perceive the relationship between aroma and colour, although this is mostly at an unconscious level. We all have a personal and intuitive relationship with aroma and colour, each of us has our favourites. Wearing perfume is one of the ways we can make a statement about who we are and how we feel about ourselves although on an intuitive level we are usually attracted to colours and aromas which are in harmony with our internal vibrations.

Aroma personalities are well understood by makers of commercial perfumes. A particular scent can conjure up an image of the person who wears it, their looks, personality and the colours they are attracted to. A well-known fashion house describes their latest perfume as being a passionate Latin, who loves the colour red. This description conjures up the aroma of rich heavy scent of Mediterranean flowers intermingled with oils and spices. So although we have an individual relationship with colour and aroma, there is also agreement that certain colours and aromas convey similar messages and share many qualities.

Although colour and aroma have a profound influence on our physical well-being, increasingly we are realising that these are not only physical forces but spiritual ones which have a profound affect on all aspects of our being.

Aroma vibrations have the capacity to by-pass the middle brain – that part of our mind which rationalises, analyses, reasons and censors our responses to the world. Like music and colour, aroma has an immediate effect on our soul, and we respond to it with our emotions and heart.

When we view ourselves as 'embodied spirits' we are reminded that we are made up of seven vibrating energetic bodies, only one of which is visible. The light and aroma generated by our internal vibrations within both the physical and spiritual dimensions connects us to each other, and also the great cosmic forces. So although aroma has physical components, it also exists in vibrational form and is conveyed through the ether to our subtle bodies.

This association of aroma with our spiritual essence has been neglected for too long and if we can rebuild this connection, it will help us regain wholeness and balance in our lives. As the essence of light and aroma exists in the fourth dimension where there is no linear time or separation of energy, the two are inextricably linked. By developing our sensitivity to them and through their synergistic healing power we have the key by which we can regain our lost sixth sense.

———————

Section One

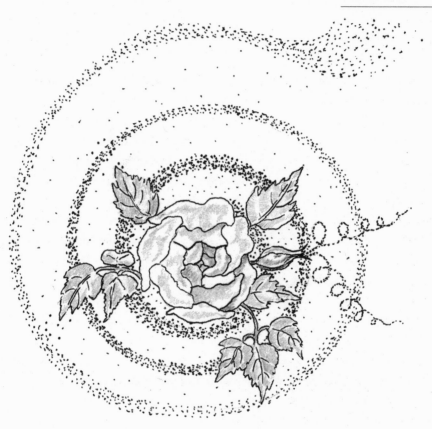

The Butterfly Effect

It was discovered by Albert Einstein in 1905 that all matter is made up from energy and that what we perceive as hard matter is mostly empty space with a pattern of energy running through it. The physical universe is really one of pure energy, and it is only the limitation of our senses which prevents us from seeing it this way.

Everything in the universe is made up of a moving mass of particles. Atoms and molecules are in a constant state of movement, creating electrical vibrations which pass from one to another. Groups of molecules vibrate at the same rate or frequency, have sympathetic resonance and these molecules are held together in groups by the frequency of their movement, forming physical matter.

In our bodies too, vibrating molecules form themselves into cells, which collect together with other cells of a sympathetic vibration and have a similar specialised function. These in turn form tissues, organs, glands and all parts of the body. All the cells communicate with one another through vibrational impulses which interchange; light, sound, aroma and electrical currents aid this exchange. These energy currents do not stop at our skin but flow between organisms so that when we meet other people there is an interchange of energy. If a person has vibrations which are in sympathetic resonance with ours, we will like them, while those people with discordant vibrations will 'get on our nerves.'

Movement of energy, no matter how small, is subject to 'The Butterfly effect'. If a butterfly flaps its wings in one part of the world eventually its effect will be felt in every part of the world no matter how distant. It is incredible to think that every movement of energy has an effect on all other living things including the mineral, plant and animal kingdom and is able to change our state of well-being at all levels.

Chain reactions of this kind stretch beyond the physical level and both colour and aroma act as catalysts for change which reach beyond the space and time where they first manifest. How many times has a bunch of red roses started a chain of romantic events, or one moment of shimmering light been the inspiration for a great artist? Many a mystical revelation has been heralded by a vision of light, the results of which have changed the lives of millions of people for generations.

In order to lead a balanced and healthy life we need to harmonise the constantly moving life-giving vibrations, allowing a flow of life-force energy (also known as prana or Ch'i) to flow freely through us. When this happens we are linked to the universal forces which pass through our system, making us feel whole and connected.

When our internal vibrations are in harmony with the world and with each other, we are healthy and have high energy levels. Our healthy state can however be affected by forced resonance from other energy systems with different frequencies. If these stronger vibrations are disharmonious they will override the existing patterns in our system causing stress and disharmony in our subtle bodies. If these discordant vibrations are not removed, illness will result.

Disease is therefore, really energetic imbalance or 'dis-ease' of our internal vibrations. Vibratory patterns have the tendency to seek equilibrium, but many times this self-levelling ability within us is not able to function due to the presence of strong vibrations which block out the natural healing patterns. Discordant vibrations can be found in the external environment but often originate in the mind or through the suppression of our emotions. This means our state of mind and our emotions greatly affects our propensity to succumb to illness.

Vibrational healing systems of which colour and aroma are a part, introduce harmonious vibrations into the system so that balance and the flow of light energy can be restored. These tune our internal vibrations, bringing the discordant vibrations back into harmony.

Nature has provided us with a perfect set of tuning tools in the plant kingdom. Plants are formed by light energy absorbed by the sun and this crystallised energy vibrates at a certain rate, holding the plant together. Plants are the perfect healers, and it is not only the actual physical plant material which sustains us in good health, but the light and aroma vibrations reflected within them. The colour and aroma vibrations held within plants set up a positive vibratory pattern in our energetic system, and through the process of resonance, set up a positive blueprint allow-ing natural healing to take place.

These pure vibrations pervade our physical body and subtle bodies, restoring the flow of life-force energy through our entire system. Where physical medicine can only affect and control our physical body, the vibrations of colour and aroma pervade and disperse energy blocked within our emotional, mental and spiritual bodies. In this way many physical ailments can be prevented before they manifest and many chronic illnesses, which appear to have no cause, can be permanently banished.

THE HEALING POWER OF COLOUR

Most people think of colour as reflected light which disappears when they close their eyes, but colour is a force which exists in its own right. Whether one is awake or asleep, sighted or blind, the coloured rays of light permeate every level of our being.

Colour vibrations come to earth in the form of light vibrations in the form of pure white sunlight which forms a part of the electro-magnetic spectrum. We can only see approximately 40% of the electro-magnetic spectrum, and this part is known to us as the visible spectrum or rainbow colours. We can compare colours to musical notes, with octaves of colours going up and down in scale and within the visible spectrum are forty octaves of colour vibrations from the darkest shades to the palest of tints.

In order to be healthy we require the energy from all the spectrum colours. Each colour vibration has a particular wave length and speed or frequency and each coloured ray has its own specific life-enhancing quality and healing action. In the visible spectrum, red is the slowest vibra-tion and has the longest wave length, while violet has the fastest vibration and shortest wave-length. Red is full of life-force energy which is reflected in the colour of our blood and our physical body, while blue connects us to the ether, linking us to our subtle bodies, and our higher mind.

Sunlight contains all the necessary elements to maintain life on earth and plants and animals have the capacity to transmute these elements into the physical and vibrational nutrition they require for health and vitality. Since the pioneering work of German educationalist and philosopher Rudolf Steiner early this century, it has become accepted that colour has a profound effect on both the mind and the body. Cells are both light sensitive and light emitting structures and when light vibration reach the cells, (via the eyes, skin and aura) fine chemical changes occur affecting their behaviour and growth. In this way the genetic and informational material of the cell (the DNA within the cell's nuclei) can be opened to healing. So, light affects us at cellular level, having a profound effect on our genetic make-up and the vibrational energy in our subtle bodies.

Each gland, body organ and body system has a sympathetic vibrational frequency as one of the rainbow colours. The cells vibrate in the same rhythmic pattern as a colour vibration and this colour vibration can be used to balance and heal that group of cells forming the tissue of an organ or gland. All our body systems move in harmony with natural rhythms, so our blood and body fluids flow in sympathy with certain wave-lengths of colour.

Colour frequency	Sympathetic gland	Sympathetic organ or body part	Body system with sympathetic frequency
Red	Adrenals	kidneys, bladder, lower limbs	muscles, blood
Orange	ovaries, testes	sexual organs, colon	digestion, lymphatic system
Yellow	pancreas	liver, gall-bladder, spleen	autonomic nervous system
Green	thymus	heart, arms	circulation, para-sympathetic nervous system
Blue	thyroid	para-thyroid, throat, ears	respiration, venous blood
Indigo	pituitary gland	eyes, nose, lower brain	skeleton, bones
Violet	pineal gland	upper brain, head	central nervous system and spine, psyche

Light also has the ability to alter our mental state by stimulating the production of certain chemicals and the central nervous system. Warming magnetic colour vibrations activate certain mental processes, while electrical colours such as blue can sedate and calm the mind. Higher frequency colour vibrations, like Indigo and Violet have a narcotic and euphoric action, and can even induce a state similar to that produced by anaesthesia. The purifying and transformative quality of violet makes it a wonderful aid to meditation.

As our cells also emit their own light vibrations, the colours reflected in our body can indicate the state of our internal environment. In Chinese medicine, body colour and odour has been used for thousands of years to reflect the condition of our state of health. The colour of the skin, eyes and tongue shows our state of health and imbalances in the energetic system can be revealed by sweet, sour, rancid, or acrid smells.

Colours are also related to the five natural elements of fire, wood, water, metal, and earth so that if the skin is red, this will reflect an imbalance of the fire element. Dark blue-black rings under the eyes will signify a problem with the urinary system and the water element. If the skin is pale, the metal element will need strengthening and yellowness of the skin and eyes reflects problems with the stomach and spleen.

In Chinese philosophy, colour was not only related to body organs and body systems, but to the fundamental energy 'Ch'i' which embodied life-giving light. A good flow of Ch'i indicated health and vitality and allowed for connection with the cosmic forces. Elemental colours are also used to harmonise the emotions and mental states which are linked to the energy flowing through the twelve energy pathways (meridians).

LIFE QUALITIES AND LESSONS OF THE RAYS

Not all light vibrations which are received through the eyes are used for the purpose of sight as colour energy has a profound effect on our metabolism. When the light vibrations enter the eye, they travel via the hypothalamus to the pituitary and the pineal glands. These master glands of the endocrine system have a powerful influence on our moods and emotions.

Each gland produces certain hormones which are released into the system, affecting the way we feel. In order for our metabolism to function normally, we need exposure to all the colour frequencies, thus providing a balance of light energy in our system. This is why it is so important we should have as much natural sunlight as possible. People who live for long periods indoors, with a lack of natural light often suffer from a range of physical, mental and emotional problems. If the pineal and pituitary do not receive a balance of every colour energy, hormone production will be inhibited or accelerated. The resulting imbalance of hormones in our body will affect our emotional stability and lead to mood swings.

On an esoteric level, colour has such a powerful effect on our emotions because it keys and activates the body's chakra system – the seven mystic energy centres running from the head to the base of the spine. These invisible power houses of the subtle etheric body each represent different aspects of being, from love to communication. Each chakra allows us to express emotions and qualities related to the individual chakras, and when energy flows we feel 'whole' and at peace with ourselves and the world. Each chakra and its related colour vibration are in turn linked to the body's major organs and glandular systems. Since each chakra is stimulated and energised by a particular colour, we can contribute significantly to our own well-being by bringing particular colours into our daily lives.

While we exist in the world of ego in our physical incarnation, we are also part of the divine world of spirit. The soul connects our dual nature, mediating between our higher mind and finer emotions and the lower mind and emotions related to our physical desires. It keeps our feet on the ground by the physical connection while allowing us to explore our spirituality.

We are at last beginning to realise that science and philosophy are coming together in their realisation that everything in the universe is evolving towards a state of perfection. Scientists believe that natural selection will produce changes in the physical body and philosophers understand that changes will also occur at deeper levels. As a binding force, the soul evolves as it moves towards increasingly higher states of consciousness. Connecting with our higher nature, through the soul, enables us to transcend the ego and embrace a loving, humble and compassionate life.

Colour exists on the physical plane, but also transcends into the spiritual realms for Divine light embodies our highest aspirations and is the purest healing force in the universe. This makes colour the perfect tool for nourishing the spirit, as the soul has a natural tendency to be drawn to the cosmic light. Each colour vibration embodies a lesson and challenge which helps our inner evolution so that we can raise our consciousness and ultimately become re-united with the divine within us. By really coming to know ourselves, we become whole and at peace with ourselves and the world.

Colour	Life-quality	Lesson or challenge
Red	self-awareness	to walk with determination on your path in life
Orange	self-respect	to enjoy creative expression and body connection
Yellow	self-worth	to find your personal power and inner radiance
Green	self-love	to trust in the abundance of nature and let love flow
Blue	self-expression	to freely express inner thoughts and feelings
Dark Blue	self-responsibility	to heighten our awareness and sensitivity to beauty and love
Violet	self-knowledge	to open oneself to one's spirituality and unity with the universe
Magenta	selflessness	to balance your own needs with needs of others.

The healing quality of each colour provides the tool which can help us meet the challenge of life's lessons. Time is meaningless when it comes to healing and wholeness. When we have learned the lesson we move on to the lesson of a higher vibration, progressing up through the spectrum. It may take us a life-time to meet one challenge, or we may be able to move up quickly through several during this life-time. We are normally attracted to the colour and aroma related to the lesson and these remain with us until we are ready to move on to the next lesson. The life-quality each brings helps us on our journey towards self-knowledge.

It is through right action that we can learn the lesson of strength to find our true purpose in life. Red energy gives us the stamina and vitality to meet this challenge. Orange energy feeds the sacral centre that links to our creative and procreative energy. By stimulating this area it warms and nourishes our emotions, so that we learn to accept and enjoy our body. This warming and releasing colour helps us release repressed emotions through creative expression especially in our relationships.

Yellow is a sunny and inspirational colour which reflects the radiance of our own inner sun. Our 'sol' or 'soul' is our seat of power and energy from the solar-plexus, radiating with golden light. Many gold flowers like daisies and sunflowers look like the sun by echoing this radial formation. Golden-yellow can nourish our soul, helping us regain our personal power.

Green is the colour of nature, and if we open our heart to nature's cycles and rhythms we will learn that there is a time and place for everything in life. Spring is the time for new growth, summer for flowering, autumn for gathering in and winter for resting. We can use the colour green to open our hearts so that abundance can come to us at the right time.

The lesson of blue is to express our thoughts and feelings with truth, trust and loyalty. Too often we are afraid of saying what we really think or believe and sublimate our true feelings for fear of criticism or rejection. Blue energy activates the throat chakra so that we can express ourselves with the voice.

The midnight blue of Indigo works through our third eye and helps us develop inner vision. The lesson of Indigo is related to heightening our sensitivity to love, truth and beauty and by so doing link to our intuition and higher mind. Once we meet the challenge of this lesson we are able to see the world with new clarity and understanding.

Violet brings with it the life-quality of self-knowledge. It is through the lesson that violet holds that we can dedicate ourselves to serving others and not just ourselves. Violet helps us disassociate ourselves from our senses, and through transformation and regeneration dissolves the feeling of separation between us and the rest of the world. So, the Violet ray promotes balance between the body, mind and spirit.

Magenta is a beautiful colour which belongs to a higher octave of colour outside our normal vision. Its fine vibration is a mixture of red and violet and it symbolises emotional balance. Magenta helps us to challenge existing structures in our lives, so that we can become mature and learn to detach ourselves from them in a loving way. The healing power of magenta helps us serve humanity in a caring and practical way, without negating our own needs.

Just as we need a variety of food to provide us with physical nutrition we also need a balance of energetic vibrations to nourish our spirit. The modern scientific use of Colour Therapy enables us to use colour to heal the body, but the ancient systems of healing with light and aroma provides us with a way of nourishing and healing our heart and soul.

COLOUR AND AROMA

We all have a personal relationship with colour and aroma, attracted to some and not to others. All these vibrations do, however, have universal qualities which affect us whether we like them or not.

For many years it has been accepted that aroma exists in chemical form, and that it is the effects of these chemicals which act as a healing agent. More recently, medical practitioners are working on the idea that the chemical messages may be passed through our body through vibrationary movements much the same as electricity is passed around the nervous system.

Now researchers into the nature and effects of aroma are coming to the conclusion that odour has two distinct forms which exist simultaneously. The first form is that of chemical molecules which can be inhaled and which penetrate our body through the skin, and the second is vibrational so that odours can affect us without any molecules reaching our nose.

If aroma exists in vibrational form, this means that every odour has a subtle vibration which can be equated to a sound and a colour and that every colour carries aromatic messages – a correspondence that has long been recognised by many ancient healing systems.

Some clairvoyant people can see the relationship between vibrations of aroma and colour and can direct colours, scents and sounds to promote inner healing. Everybody can develop their own sensitivity to these vibrations, and there are many ways to develop our inner senses so that we can experience the relationship between particular aromas and colours. If we also understand the actions and the healing qualities of these vibrations we can direct them through our energetic field by introducing a healing agent, such as a flower essence or essential oil.

Some people, like the American researcher R.H. White, take a more scientific approach in finding the connections between colour and aroma. He uses thermodynamics as grounds for comparing the vibrations of odours with the electro-magnetic spectrum. As odour is invisible, he draws the conclusion that aromatic vibrations fall outside the visible spectrum and must therefore correspond with the infra-red part of the spectrum. What White fails to do is to find the correspondence between odours and visible colours and other areas of the colour spectrum.

It makes sense that if aroma vibrations exist in the longer wave lengths of the electro-magnetic spectrum, they should also exist through the visible spectrum to the higher wave lengths. We know that colour and aroma overlap on the physical plane, because babies and some adults experience aromas as visible colours and are able to physically smell colours. Complementary practitioners and their patients often report experiencing colours when giving or receiving treatments. So it seems that aroma is linked to colour through many octaves, from the invisible long waves, through the visible spectrum to the invisible short wave frequencies.

INTUITIVE COLOURS

We often sense the relationship between colours and fragrances intuitively. This happens when we are doing something which does not involve our usual daily mental processes. When we do everyday tasks, we are using the left side of our brain and lower mind which is concerned with logic, order, planning, language and other cognitive skills. It is only when we connect with our right hand brain and higher mind, that we access our intuition and experience vibrational connections beyond our normal perception. The right side of the brain is more abstract and free to exercise creative, emotional, empathetic and spontaneous interaction with the universe.

Through techniques such as colour breathing, creative visualisation and meditation, we can disconnect from the constant chatter of the lower mind. We can also connect with our intuition when the lower mind is occupied. By focussing on a task, it enables us to become aware of impulses coming from the soul. Many therapists experience synthesis while giving an holistic treatment, as it is also through empathy and love that we become receptive to subtle forces around us. The third most common way we experience vibrational connections is while we enjoy the freedom of movement in our astral body while we sleep. When we move without restrictions of space and time we can joyously tune in to vibrational harmonies.

Our intuitive knowledge of the links between colour and aroma is impossible to analyse, as there are an infinite number and combination of colours and aromas we may experience. It may be that different relationships mean different things at different times and so I think it is important to accept these moments of enlightenment without judgement or analysis. If you are aware of certain colours while working with a flower or aromatic oil, and you feel a person needs a certain colour energy at that moment, direct it to them through your hands, or open heart chakra. By the same token if you are working with colour and you get a strong urge to use a specific aroma for healing, follow that path without question.

We can direct positive vibrations spontaneously at this unconscious level, but it is by heightening our awareness and bringing spirit into matter that transmutation necessary for permanent healing occurs. Stagnant or blocked energy must be moved from the unconscious to the conscious in order for it to be recognised, accepted and dissipated. This is the basis of vibrational healing.

VIBRATIONAL HEALING

Whilst we can see many colours that are in the lower wave-lengths of light, there are many colours in higher octaves that vibrate at such a level as to be visible only through inner vision. Similarly, some aromas have a frequency and sympathetic vibration to visible colours, while other aromas have such a high frequency that they harmonise with colour vibrations well outside our normal visible colour range. Most of us only get a glimpse of these when we connect with our intuition by withdrawing from the outer world and going within ourselves.

In order to work with colour and aroma we need to reduce this infinite number of vibrations to those within our sensory range so that we have a tangible tool for healing. Colour vibrations progress up the electro-magnetic scale in octaves, in the same way as musical notes rise in pitch. If we know odour corresponds to the invisible wave-lengths of the electro-magnetic spectrum, by linking aroma to the visible rainbow we have to change the frequency of the vibrations, so it falls within our sensory range.

By changing the harmonies of aroma to the visible spectrum, the resonance remains in the same harmonic. This is similar to playing the same tune on a piano at a higher key. The tune will remain the same although the pitch will be changed.

We can use this melody to set up harmonious vibrations in our body, mind and spirit, knowing that we will also be directing finer vibrations of aroma and colour to our system.

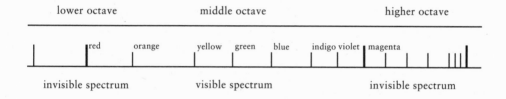

Electro-magnetic spectrum

Although we cannot see either true white nor true magenta, I have included both these colours into the healing spectrum. True magenta is a mixture of infra-red and ultra-violet light both of which are invisible to our eyes. We do, however, see a wonderful approximation of magenta in many beautiful flowers which have an iridescent quality to them. White cannot be considered as a colour as it has no density and merely reflects all the colours of the spectrum. Some flowers do appear white, although on closer examination, most of them are a very pale tint of another colour.

The vibrations produced by our bodies are too dense to respond to the true healing power of white light and it is for this reason we need to break down white light into its colour components which vibrate at lower frequencies. These slower rainbow colours are more effective in moving energy blocks in the subtle bodies thus allowing life-giving white light to flow unobstructed through our system. The finer energy in our spiritual bodies is especially receptive to the healing qualities reflected in the aroma and colour of White flowers.

The colours and aromas sympathetic to the middle frequencies of visible light are not only pleasurable to our senses; they affect us at an emotional level. These vibrations of colours and aroma are in tune with our inner energetic vibrations and thus heal us at a deeper level.

If we are to make use of this infinite source of energy, we need to bring it down to earth and find a form which embodies harmonious elements of colour and aroma vibrations. It is through the plant kingdom that we can find the perfect solution. Nature has provided us with plants for our physical and vibrational sustenance and not only do these medicines contain the right contents, they are also packaged with aromatic and colour labelling which indicates their exact properties. By learning to read these markers we have at our disposal a divine encyclopaedia of colour and aroma relationships.

For most people wishing to use a tangible tool, we need to use a healing agent, which contains colour and aroma as an integral part. Essential oils provide this wonderful medium whereby we can combine both these vibrations into our system.

The aroma molecules in essential oils enter our body through our skin, causing chemical reactions occur which bring about physical, emotional and mental changes. On a vibrational level, different oils have affinities with different parts of the body which have a natural sympathetic reson-ance. Like colour, the aroma vibrations permeate our aura and work on our etheric body through the chakra system and the network of energetic meridians.

Often it is the vibrations we do not like that we need to restore energetic balance. We all know that often we avoid food which is good for us, knowingly basing our diet on that which has little nutritional con-tent which could ultimately damage our health. This rejection of certain vibrations can prove difficult for a therapist wishing to give a healing treatment.

The sympathetic resonance of aroma and colour provide a good solution for if you have an aversion to a particular aroma you can introduce the corresponding colour vibration, while a dislike for a certain colour could be balanced with the introduction of an aroma with an affinity to that colour. It is a matter of finding the right form of the vibration which is acceptable to one. For instance, if you find the colour green abhorrent, you could introduce Geranium oil into your energetic system to restore balance, while the use of Red can be substituted if you detest the aroma of Jasmine.

COLOUR AND AROMA IN THE AURA

Not only do we experience the colours in our surroundings visually and respond to odour through our sense of smell, we also absorb their vibrational energy through our aura.

The aura acts as a prism through which vital white light energy passes. The light is broken down into its component colours and sent to energise the individual energy centres or 'chakras'. It is only when light energy, containing all the colours, flows uninterrupted through us, connecting us to the cosmic forces, that we can be in perfect health and enjoy harmony in our life.

Just as the earth is surrounded and protected by the ozone layer, our aura filters vibrations from the outside world. Colours and aromas from our surroundings are absorbed into our aura and permeate our energetic system which flows around our system in a network of invisible energy lines much like the ley-lines running through the earth. In a strong healthy individual the aura provides protection encircling us with a strong force field of electro-magnetic energy. If there is disharmony or imbalance in our system, the aura will become depleted allowing harmful vibrations in. If the aura is not energised, holes will appear as they have done in the earth's ozone layer and the breaks need to be plugged and energy flow restored.

Essential oils and colours can re-charge the aura, while others can cleanse the negative vibrations from the subtle bodies. It is then possible to set up positive vibrations to seal and heal the auric field.

Magenta/Red	energises the force field	Rosemary, Clary Sage
Blue	heals the auric field	Juniper, Sandalwood
Violet/White	purifies and seals the aura	Lavender, Frankincense

15

While vibrations from the outside world permeate our aura, the flow is not only inwards. The aura also contains light and sound vibrations emitted by all our physical and etheric cells, glands and organs. Our state of health and our state of consciousness is reflected by the array and proportions of colour and aroma vibrations in our aura.

People who are filled with vitality and good health exude clear bright colours and are surrounded by a sweet smelling aroma, while those people who have energy blocked within their system will be surrounded by darker colours and a less pleasant aroma. Various types of Aura photography and those people with clairvoyant vision, have revealed that bodies polluted by smoke, drink and drugs display muddy and murky browns and blacks in their aura, and we all know that these people also exude a bad odour.

Our favourite colours and aromas reveal the quality of the vibrations in our aura, as we are attracted to vibrations which are in harmony with our own. Although the colours in our mental and emotional bodies are constantly changing, the quality and tone of these vibrations stays constant for most of our lives. The lightness, brightness of the colours and note of the aroma indicates our state of consciousness, including our personality traits, qualities and lessons to be learned this life-time.

An attraction to new colours or scent usually reveals an unconscious search for the vibrations which are required to balance and heal some part of our being where there is disharmony. These colours can help us understand ourselves better.

Everyone has good and bad qualities, strengths and weaknesses. Colour too is neither good nor bad, for each colour energy displays positive and negative aspects and it is only when we have a colour energy imbalance in our system that we tend to display the negative aspects of a colour. It may be that you have too much of one colour energy and too little of another. If you find you are displaying the negative qualities of green, you need to add some red into your life. The positive motivation that red provides will help alleviate such problems as lethargy, depression or indecisiveness.

Colour and aroma are excellent tools for balancing the emotions and encouraging positive personality traits. Use this guide to your colours and the related oils to help you attract their positive qualities. You can introduce the colours into your daily life and through an aromatherapy massage or colour treatment.

Colour	Personality	Positive quality	Negative quality
Red	outgoing, active, physical	motivated, warm, stable, strong	irritability, anger, impatience
Orange	sociable, creative	practical, joyful, assimilating, expressive	over-stimulating, tiring, sexual excess
Yellow	quick alert mind, sunny, ideas	bright, happy, logical, communicative	egocentric, fearful, critical
Green	caring, empathetic, natural	balance, harmony, abundance, flexible, aspiration	indecisive, feeling trapped
Blue	peaceful, quiet, introverted	loyal, honesty, direct, adaptable	depressive, withdrawn, lacking trust
Purple	creative, spiritual, sensitive	powerful, seeker of truth, inspirational	misuse of power, obsessive, addictive
Peach	warm, caring	creative, supportive, charitable, mature	sentimental, low self-esteem
Pink	loving, nurturing, emotional	understanding, sympathetic	immature, needy, emotionally unstable
Turquoise	fresh, sparkle, new ideas	uplifting, refreshing, communicative, cool	cold, isolating, over-sensitive
Pastels	softer version of each colour	more sensitive, gentle	easily led, impressionable

OUR SUBTLE BODIES

Unlike the physical body whose vibrations are slow and dense and therefore visible to us, the subtle bodies vibrate at a quicker rate and are invisible to ocular sight. Even though these radiant bodies are invisible, the energy of the physical and radiant bodies is interconnected as a relationship of exchange and mutual influence exists between all our bodies. It is the rate of vibration which is the central difference between the physical and radiant bodies. This difference of vibration extends to the world of colour.

The aura is made up a several discernible layers of energy which surround the physical body spreading outwards to form an egg shape. The first layer of the aura is made up of the vibrations from both the physical body and the physical duplicate known as the etheric body. On the etheric level this energy can be perceived as a pale red light becoming more intense where there is good vitality and a strong force field. This red colouring reveals the ability and flow of the basic life force in the individual and permeates out from the base chakra. The physical body connects with the base chakra and the colour red, while a lighter version of red, deep rose pink, pervades the etheric body.

More often we are aware of the etheric energy around someone when we feel the tingle of electricity coming from them. The etheric body has organs, tissues and cells exactly the same as the physical body, but the nervous system in the etheric body is known as the meridian system. This system of energy lines permeates the etheric body in much the same way as the nerve network of the physical body with which it is strongly linked. Any changes that occur in the energy of the meridians directly affects the nervous system.

Like colour, odour is a vibration which travels in the ether thus affecting our etheric body and its effects on this subtle level will also be interpreted by the physical body. Good vibrations will manifest as good health, while disharmonious vibrations will result in illness.

The second layer in the aura comprises the radiation from the emotional body and is linked to energy in the sacral and throat chakras. The colours and shapes in this layer show our changing moods as well as our general emotional health. This layer is also known as the astral body. Within the second layer is found the mental body, which is permeated with our thought waves, positive and negative. In this layer we can see our mind waves and the more set patterns of thought created over a long period of time. The mental body has two distinct bands, that of the lower mind, consisting of energy coming from the solar-plexus, and that from the higher mind which flows to and from the heart centre.

The third layer is made up of several bands of spiritual bodies, which may extend many metres around us depending on our spiritual development. This part of the aura may reveal beautiful colours and exquisite aromas which can only be seen during meditation or by those with clairvoyant vision. The heart centre, which is the seat of the soul, also connects with the spiritual bodies as well as the brow and crown chakras.

When working with essential oils and colour vibrations we need to become sensitive to the colours and aromas in the aura. Often you will be able to tune in to the colours needed by you or someone else and channel these vibrations through your hands. The more you work with subtle energy the easier it becomes to develop the ability to blend oils intuitively. It is, however, most important that we have a sound knowledge of the therapeutic qualities and actions of both colour energy and essential oil vibrations, for healing intuitively can be very dangerous if practised by someone without a sound understanding of the powerful effects they can have on us.

HEALING THROUGH THE ETHERIC

It is through the medium of the etheric plane that we can bring spirit into matter, and so it is not by accident that we can influence both our physical and spiritual being, by introducing healing vibrations of colour and aroma into the etheric body.

When we look at our energetic make-up as a whole we will see that the etheric body is pivotal. Every cell, tissue and organ in the physical body has an etheric counterpart, like a secret partner. Energy flows around the physical body like an electric current which is generated by the brain, and sent down the nerves of the central autonomic and sympathetic nervous system. In the etheric the counterpart network of energy carriers is known as the meridian system, which spreads throughout the etheric body in the same way. The energy circulating around the etheric body cannot be detected by normal vision because it exists in a higher plane which is beyond our sensory perception.

The physical and etheric body is so closely connected that the physical body mirrors everything on the etheric level but interprets the image in a physical way. The etheric body also acts as a funnel, collecting energy gathered from the subtle bodies and directing it to the physical body.

Healthy vibrations in the etheric are interpreted as good health and vitality by the physical body, while imbalance and distorted energy in the etheric will be interpreted as illness and disease.

The radiation patterns and energy field given off by the etheric body can be captured on film, through the process known as Kirlian photography. Kirlian photography can be very useful to a complementary healer to show the difference between energy levels before and after a treatment. Aura photography which is a growing field also reveals colourful bands of energy in the emotional and mental body but cannot pick up the fine vibrations in the spiritual bodies.

Within our etheric body we have seven energy centres, known as chakras, which are spaced at intervals from the base of the spine to the top of our head and joined along the spine. Each chakra affects the energy levels and workings of specific body organs and glands as well as certain systems in the body.

Each chakra needs a balance of all the colour vibrations, but the individual chakras are also tuned in to a particular colour vibration, much the same way as a radio receiver. The organs and glands connected to the chakra will also be tuned in to this colour wave-length. When there is disharmony in our being, whether it be physically, emotionally, mentally or spiritually, one or more of our energy centres can lose its signal. Just as a radio channel loses its station, the chakra needs to be re-tuned so that it can once again receive the colour signal loud and clear. We can do this by introducing the appropriate colour until harmony is restored. Essential oils which have a sympathetic frequency with a particular chakra reinforce the action. So we can adjust the energy levels in the etheric before any negative vibrations reach the physical body. By introducing colour energy we can open, energise and free the flow of energy through the chakras.

COLOUR KEYS TO ENERGISING THE CHAKRAS

1. RED   The lowest centre located at the base of the spine
2. ORANGE   The splenic centre in the small of the back.
3. YELLOW   The middle of the back, solar plexus.
4. GREEN   The heart centre in between the shoulder blades.

5.	TURQUOISE	The thymus gland in the middle of the upper chest (minor chakra)
6.	BLUE	The throat or thyroid at the base of the skull.
7.	INDIGO	The third eye, the pineal gland.
8.	VIOLET	The crown of the head, pituitary gland.
9.	WHITE	Just above the crown of the head

Essential oils also have an affinity with certain chakras, which they benefit. The lower chakras which relate to the physical body and are strongly connected to earth energy, can be stimulated and energised by oils vibrating on the red ray. Most of these oils contain magnetic earth energy and are made from Yang parts of the plant, that is the roots or stem. They might also be related due to the colour of the flowers or seeds. Using these associated oils on the chakra areas along the spine or on the foot reflex, can help balance the chakra to which the oil is linked. Thus aroma and colour vibrations can work together to balance and heal every part of our being through the chakra system.

THE HEALING ACTIONS AND QUALITIES OF COLOURS

The universe is perfectly organised, whole, where nothing happens without reason and everything is moving towards a definite goal. In living things this continuous state of evolution takes place on both the physical and spiritual plane simultaneously. So while our body adapts and evolves to the environment, our consciousness is also moving towards a state of perfection. Illness is therefore the consequence of disharmony within the cosmic order ruled by the universal law of cause and effect, often known as Karma. Disharmony within us cannot be reduced to individual parts, and in order for us to restore balance, the body, mind and soul must be considered integral.

The healing power of light provides us will all the elements we require to keep all parts of our being in good health but in order to make use of the therapeutic qualities of colour vibrations we need to understand their actions upon our physical and subtle bodies. Modern medicine already makes use of many of the invisible wave lengths of light but for the most part these can be highly dangerous and invasive practices. Laser beams are being used more and more for surgery although these longer wave-lengths destroy healthy and diseased cells and tissue indiscriminately. While the powerful rays of visible light are unable to blast away matter in a dramatic way, they are still powerful enough move and disperse energy through our whole system, restoring harmony with the least shock or disruption.

There are of course hundreds of colour variations which we can use for healing purposes and so it is practical to use only the rainbow colours and a few colours in a higher octave which are still visible to the human eye. These lighter vibrations have a similar effect to the pure hue from which they are derived but as they contain more white light, they are gentler in their action and more pervasive on our subtle bodies.

Darker tones reflect less light and through forced resonance, have a stronger and more direct effect on our energetic system. These tones are useful for dealing with physical problems and will influence our emotions, especially at times when immediate action is required. Pale blue will have a similar effect as pure blue, while lavender will reflect the softer qualities of the violet ray.

Flowers, herbs and essential oils have a sympathetic harmonic to different colour wave-lengths. When considering the colour frequency of an essential oil, we need to decide whether it reflects the pure rainbow colour or a lighter or darker hue. An oil reflecting a pale creamy-yellow will have different qualities from one containing rich golden-yellow energy.

The lighter oil will have a more subtle effect, reaching the finer vibrations of the spiritual bodies, while the brighter colour will be more effective in energising the physical and etheric bodies (chakras). If you are an aromatherapist it can be useful to think of these tones of colour as different notes. The lighter colours will reflect top notes while the darker tones will reflect base notes.

RED

Base Chakra
Healing action: warming, energising, moving
Life qualities: survival, action, will

RED is the colour of life, as it is the colour of blood. By strengthening the blood, and energy in the liver and kidneys, it brings with it physical strength and stamina so that we can have vitality and good health. You will need red energy when you are tired, listless, run-down or depressed. Red stimulates the circulation of Ch'i through all the chakras bringing a state of self-awareness and presence in the physical body. The lesson of red relates to motivation, walking purposefully on our path in life and its earth connection strengthens our whole system through the base chakra. Red energy helps to ground you if you are a person who has your head in the clouds and helps us turn our ideas into action.

Physical   Connects you to primal energy, stimulates the adrenals and blood supply to the brain, activates the sexual organs and raises the pulse and heart beat. Promotes heat in the body, and the production of healthy red blood cells which is good if you are anaemic. It increases mobility where there are blocks resulting in paralysis.

Emotional Brings excitement of sensual physical love.

Mental   Gives a purpose in living, helps you take action, and strengthens your will.

Spiritual   Helps you walk on your path in life, use for chronic blockages in the energy system. Action brings with it new life.

Essential oils which reflect the Red ray:
Black Pepper, Cedarwood, Jasmine, Benzoin, Sage, Camphor (white), Myrrh, Rose, Thyme (red)

PINK
Heart Chakra
Healing action: warms and uplifts emotions,muscle relaxant
Life quality: allows the flow of love

DEEP ROSE PINK is the colour of unconditional love and is a softer version of the red. As pink is red mixed with white light, it has a gently stimulating effect on our whole system and is especially comforting and uplifting to the emotions. Rose Pink is particularly good for treating emotional problems and balancing the female aspect within us as pink links strongly to the heart chakra which must be open if we are to link to our intuition and our higher mind. Just as a pink rose is surrounded by green leaves, pink works in harmony with the colour green, to stimulate the flow of love which will attract abundance and contentment. Paler pink brings comfort and security to children and helps nurture the 'inner child' in adults.

Physical   Pink gently warms and aids circulation without raising blood pressure and is especially useful in treating the young, old or weak. Pink nourishes the feminine energy in our system and affects creativity, sex and conception.

Emotional Warming and nurturing to the emotions, provides gentle loving vibrations which can aid grieving, loss, rejection and promote self love and softens a hard heart.

Mental   Uplifts the mind by warming the emotions.

Spiritual   Promotes the ability to give and receive unconditional love.

Essential oils which reflect the Pink ray:
Rose, Rosewood, Melissa, Palmarosa, Geranium, Verbena, Jasmine, Ylang Ylang, Garlic, Eucalyptus, Cumin, Caraway, Coriander (these last three have yellow and pink vibrations)

ORANGE
Sacral chakra
Healing action: warms, opening, tonifying, releasing
Life quality: sexuality, joy and creative expression

Orange is a beautiful colour which is a mixture of red and yellow and full of radiance. While having the strength and movement of red, it is moderated by the yellow of the mind. So the orange vibration aids practicality, for we need to think before we act. Orange connects to the sacral centre which activates the sexual organs and is the energy centre which relates to our ability to find creative expression. When our sacral centre is energised we are in touch with our body enabling us to develop self-confidence and self-respect. This sensual and earthy connection enables us to move gracefully and with poise. The warmth of Orange and release afforded by this vibration promotes movement and flow through the body and emotions. Its freeing action promotes movement of all body fluids including the blood, lymph, sexual fluids and tears. Its vitality is a wonderful anti-depressant and the life-quality it promotes is one of joy and generosity.

Physical Governs the sexual organs, releases all body fluids, and activates the lymphatic system. It is a powerful tonic and increases sexual potency. Builds up the immune system and promotes the absorption of calcium.

Emotional Freeing action on the emotions helping you to release stagnant energy you are holding caused by repressed emotions from past relationships. Aids self-confidence and self-esteem.

Mental Stimulating effect of red with analytical quality of yellow, makes orange a very creative colour, but one with a practical application. It can help creative blocks. Anti-depressant.

Spiritual It is the colour of joy, good health and creativity. It charges and replenishes the aura

Essential oils which reflect the Orange ray:
Aniseed, Caraway, Ginger, Carrot Seed, Bergamot, Pine, Mandarin, Marigold (Calendula officinalis), Neroli, Nutmeg, Orange, Patchouli, Pimento, Sandalwood, Cardamon, Benzoin, Cedarwood, Cinnamon, Marjoram and Cypress (contain both orange and blue colour vibrations)

YELLOW
Solar-plexus
Healing action: strengthens mind and nervous system, cleansing
Life quality: personal power, aspiration

GOLDEN-YELLOW is the colour of the sun and is a happy and uplifting colour. On a physical level, yellow energy links to the nervous system, liver and gallbladder. It is the colour of the Christ light and the Hara centre (just below the navel), which brings with it true wisdom when working with an open heart centre. Yellow is the colour of the mind and the ego and as it links to the left-hand side of the brain it promotes logic, language skills, memory, organisation and other logical processes. It also has an affinity to the lower mind which develops patterns of thought often ingrained from childhood. Often we hold nervousness and worry in the solar-plexus, the chakra which is linked to the colour yellow, and by energising this centre with golden-yellow we regain our personal power and dispel our fears. When yellow takes on a golden hue it changes its affinity to the right-hand brain, and the higher mind. It is through our higher mind that we can develop discrimination, integrity and wisdom beyond the restrictions of our ego and then our solar-plexus glows with the radiance of our own inner sun.

Physical   Yellow has a cleansing and laxative action. It strengthens the nervous system and muscles, including the heart creating better circulation. Aids secretion of gastric juices and digestion. Helps with assimilation and elimination processes and has an alkalising effect. Aids the functioning of the liver, gall-bladder and pancreas which it stimulates to produce insulin.

Emotional   Uplifting colour, bringing hope and light and a feeling that everything will be all right. Dispels fears and nervousness and helps you develop personal power and the ability to value yourself.

Mental   Yellow is a cerebral stimulant, aiding mental clarity and concentration. It promotes open-mindedness and aids communication of thoughts. Calmness and stability of the mind can be achieved through nourishment of the central nervous system.

Spiritual   Golden-yellow brings wisdom in your affairs, signifies high ideals and helps re-charge the aura so it is protected from psychic attack.

Essential oils which reflect the Yellow ray:
Bergamot, Birch, Cardamom, Celery, Coriander, Cajeput, Citronella, Cumin, Lemon, Lemongrass, Marigold (Tagetes minuta), Grapefruit, Basil, Fennel, Vetivert, Cinnamon, Camphor (Yellow), Angelica, Aniseed, Caraway, Cedarwood, Carrot Seed, Dill, Ginger, Sandalwood (contains violet and yellow vibrations) Tea-Tree (contains indigo and yellow vibrations) Oregano, Parsley, Petitgrain, Niaouli (all contain yellow-green vibrations)

GREEN
Heart chakra
Healing action: relaxing, balancing, normalising
Life qualities: communion with nature trust in the process of life, justice

Green is nature's healing colour. It balances and harmonises our system on all levels and is wonderful for the treatment of shock and all types of stress. On a physical level it promotes harmony within our cells and has a regulating effect on our metabolism. It also has antiseptic and disinfectant qualities which cleanse us of impurities on the physical, emotional and mental level. Green is the colour associated with the heart chakra and is usually complimented with pink light to promote the flow of love and abundance. The lesson of green is to learn to trust the process of life for everything has a time and a place and you cannot rush things along. Green can provide physical and emotional space, giving you time to breathe and just be. The balancing effect green has on the pituitary gland and on our emotions, makes it excellent for the treatment of mood swings and for those wishing to regain balance in their lives.

Physical   Works on the digestive system and balances the blood pressure. It works through the sympathetic nervous system to aid relaxation and helps eliminate toxic material from the system. Balancing force for shock and is cooling for headaches. Aids normal tissue growth and helps recuperation and healing of fractures.

Emotional Stabilises extreme emotions, gives us a feeling of space and time to relax and not be pressured. Promotes sharing and empathy with others and helps develop unconditional love. Deep Rose Pink is the colour of unconditional love, and promotes the ability to give and receive love.

Mental   Provides time to let things happen naturally without forcing any issues or having to make decisions. Has a strong sedative effect and allows the conscious mind to rest.

Spiritual Balances and harmonises the aura and helps connection to the devic and spiritual realms.

Essential oils which reflect the Green ray:
Eucalyptus, Geranium, Silver Fir, Lime, Linden Blossom, Peppermint, Petitgrain, Origanum, Parsley, Star Anise, Thyme (Red), Verbena, Rosewood, Palmarosa, Melissa (pink and green vibrations) Bergamot, Celery, Marigold and Lemon (green and yellow vibrations), Bay Laurel (indigo and green vibrations), Violet (violet and green vibrations)

TURQUOISE
Thymus chakra
Healing actions: cleansing, refreshing, revitalising
Life qualities: communication, heals heart through verbal expression,
adaptability

It is not strange that there should be a resurgence of interest in turquoise as our thymus gland and the minor chakra to which it belongs becomes more active. Turquoise is made up of a mixture of blue and green, and is a cooling and refreshing colour without being static. Its therapeutic action on the body is as an acid tonic. It embodies the qualities of bubbling spring water for it is fresh and clear, and has extra sparkle. It is a colour of communication and helps us listen to and express the messages coming from the heart. Turquoise is a cerebral depressant, so that while the conscious mind is sedated, it allows connection with the impulses from the higher mind and the soul. Turquoise is an important healing colour for our times, as its relationship with the thymus gland enables it to boost the bodies own defences. It is not surprising therefore that turquoise has been found to be the favourite colour of people suffering from problems related to a depleted immune system. The close association of the thymus gland to the heart also makes the turquoise ray helpful in promoting self-love and through loving vibrations aiding our connection with the Divine.

Physical   Stimulates the thymus to make helper T-cells essential to the immune system. Useful for all inflammatory conditions, headaches, swellings, cuts and bruises. Good for skin problems caused by stress and nervous tension. Promotes a healthy immune system.

Emotional Replenishes the emotions where you are worn out by long emotional trauma. Lifts and encourages inner communication to solve relationship problems.

Mental   Promotes alertness and awareness which gives great clarity of expression. It brings open-mindedness and refreshing ideas. Good for mental exhaustion.

Spiritual   Purity of spirit and links the earth to the ethereal. Charges the thymus chakra and strengthens the etheric body.

Essential oils which reflect the Turquoise ray:
Myrtle, Niaouli, Bay Laurel (indigo and green)

BLUE
Throat Chakra
Healing action: cooling, soothing, sedating, promotes healing
Life qualities: Intuition, loyalty, truth, purity of word

BLUE is the colour of oxygen which surrounds Mother earth and also of Father sky, reminding us that we belong to both the physical and spiritual realm. Peace is always connected with blue, and it is the colour of loyalty, truth and hope. Blue is the colour chosen to represent the medical profession and it is this caring, healing quality coupled with knowledge and under-standing, that embodies blue energy. It is a very healing colour as it soothes and calms the mind and cools our systems and helps boost the body's own healing mechanism. The most important therapeutic quality of blue is pain relief, for it cools, soothes and heals. Blue helps us listen to the messages coming from our intuition, and promotes sensitivity to beauty and the creative arts. As blue has an affinity with the throat chakra, it cleanses and purifies our words so that we desire to speak well of others. The lesson of blue is to learn to trust your intuition and to take responsibility for oneself.

Physical   Anti-bacterial qualities. Releases tension headaches, sore throats, reduces fevers, inflammations, sunstroke. Treats period pains, backache and eye troubles. Good for children's ailments and eases pain of circulatory blockages. Relieves pain (although you need to treat the problem at source)

Emotional   Promotes the ability to express your feelings vocally, and the appreciation of truth, beauty and peace. Helps creative expression.

Mental   Brings inner calm to the mind and links one to one's intuition and higher self.

Spiritual   Promotes gentleness of spirit and sensitivity. Heals the etheric and mends breaks in the aura so that deep inner healing can take place.

Essential oils which reflect the Blue ray:
German Chamomile, Roman Chamomile, Myrtle, Marjoram, Thyme (White), Rosemary, Hyssop, Cypress, Pine, Mandarin (all have orange and blue vibrations), Eucalyptus (some varieties)

DEEP BLUE
Third Eye
Healing action: pain healer, anaesthetic, mind relaxant, cooling
Life quality: knowledge with understanding, purification, intuition

This DEEP BLUE is not as dark as indigo being more a royal blue and this shade of blue creates a strong cloak of maternal protection. The Virgin Mary was always depicted in a royal blue cloak, which is a similar tone to the blue found in the aura of a nursing mother. Mothers have a lot of blue in their aura, and their babies draw in the blue vibrations until their 'ego' develops as their psyche separates from the mother. Deep blue in the aura of a man may signify a protective nature, and you need to discover what they are protecting. The midnight blue of Indigo helps raise our sensitivity to the sacredness in all things, and it can be used for deep pain, healing and purification. The affinity indigo blue has with the third eye chakra brings with it clarity of vision. Rather than heightening our awareness, deep blue allows us to take responsibility and direct our thoughts, desires and energy to areas which will promote self-development and spiritual growth.

Physical   Cools the system and is a deep pain healer. Good for treatment of burns, sunstroke, itchy skin, rashes, boils. Builds up new bone tissue.

Emotional Encourages communication with the feminine aspect, and softer side of our nature, spontaneous, loving and joyful. Helps us see the beauty around us.

Mental   It is a good sedative and can produce states similar to anaesthesia. Links to the higher mind with intuition with power and knowledge.

Spiritual Protects the aura and promotes inner vision through the Third eye.

Essential oils which reflect the Indigo ray:
Bay Laurel, Clove, Tea-tree (also Turquoise ray), Yarrow, Pimento, Myrtle, Cinnamon (orange, yellow and indigo vibrations)

VIOLET
Crown Chakra
Healing action: normalising, purifying, balancing to the mind and psyche
Life quality: transformation, spirituality

VIOLET has always been associated with the spirit in religions as well as the power of kings and royalty. This is the colour of self-knowing which is very powerful. People who display a great deal of violet in their aura are seeking spiritual development and are very sensitive souls. They are likely to be highly creative but they should be careful lest they misuse the power that this colour gives them. Violet vibrates at a very high frequency and its transformative power helps dissolve fears of the mind. Its power to help us stand back from our senses allows us to strengthen our cosmic connections which ultimately brings us peace and inner harmony. Use violet to cleanse a room of impure thoughts and emotions. Violet contains both red and blue vibrations which harmonise the base and crown chakra, and on a physical level it is gently stimulating without being inflammatory.

Violet is a colour of protection for its high resonance creates a strong force field of protection through which lower psychic entities and mind waves cannot penetrate.

Physical   Normalises glandular and hormonal activity. Relieves problems in the head, ears, and nose and strengthens weak eyes. It is a blood purifier and assists with building up white blood cells. Helps treat varicose veins and anywhere stimulation is needed in inflamed or painful conditions.

Emotional   Works on the brain through the central nervous system, so is used for healing all mental and nervous disorders and personality imbalances. Harmonises the heart with the higher mind.

Mental   Promotes dignity, self-respect and tolerance. Promotes creativity and service to others. Hypnotic and narcotic effect, so sedates the mind.

Spiritual   Promotes spiritual growth. Purges, cleanses, protects and transforms the auric layers through regeneration of harmonious vibrations.

Essential oils which reflect the Violet ray:
Juniper, Lavender, Frankincense, Niaouli (also yellow and turquoise ray), Sage (Spanish), Violet, Peppermint, Hyssop, Birch, Cajuput, Carrot Seed, Grapefruit, Basil, Patchouli, Sandalwood

MAGENTA
Base and Crown
Healing actions: nourishing, energising, harmonises emotions and
higher mind
Life qualities: co-operation and service

MAGENTA is made up of a mixture of violet and red and belongs to a
higher octave of colour. This makes magenta a very high healing
frequency and a unifying and balancing light vibration. The red part of it
provides stimulation and strength, while the violet part contains blue
which is soothing and sedating. Magenta is a cardiac energiser, especially
useful for stimulating movement of arterial and venous blood where
there is swelling, inflammation or heat in the body. It also stimulates the
adrenals and supra-renals, both glands which activate the flow of life-
force energy through our system. On an emotional level, magenta
promotes a mature attitude to life, service to others and spirituality while
being practical and well grounded. The red in magenta provides us with
purpose and stamina and lifts the vibrations in the base chakra. The violet
directs us along a spiritual path so we can find peace and fulfilment.

Physical	Use to promote strength and the flow of blood without increasing the heart beat. It boosts life-force energy (Ch'i) especially in states of collapse and unconsciousness
Emotional	Promotes emotional maturity by balancing your own needs with those of others
Mental	Transformative to the mind, so you can see life from another perspective
Spiritual	Stimulates the flow of Ch'i through all the chakras. Learning spiritual lessons through dreamwork

Essential oils which reflect the Magenta ray:
Ylang Ylang, Clary Sage

WHITE
Over Crown
Healing actions: purifying emotions, cleansing of spirit, auric protection
Life qualities: state of grace, enlightenment

WHITE is the colour of pure sunlight which contains all the other colours. Its high vibrations have a cleansing and purifying action on us, working through the crown chakra and activating life force energy (Ch'i) through all our chakras. For most people their own vibrations are too slow to be sensitive to the healing qualities of white light and this is why we usually direct the healing qualities of the coloured components for healing. For some people who are extremely sensitive, such as some mediums, healers, artists and musicians and those following a spiritual path, white light can be used directly for healing. We can all, however, benefit from the healing rays in natural sunlight by spending as much time as possible in natural light, as well as making use of the light vibrations captured in plants. White light embodied in flowers helps us on our path to discovering truth, stillness and inner vision.

Physical   Stimulating the flow of Ch'i through all the chakras-raising energy levels

Emotional   Cleansing and purifying action on the emotions

Mental   Liberating and releasing of negative thought patterns and connection with the unconscious and higher mind.

Spiritual   Purification of the spirit allowing for soul growth by connecting the flow of love energy from the heart. Opens the crown chakra so we can connect with universal light and experience the state of grace.

Essential oils which reflect the White ray:
Carnation, Narcissus, Gardenia, Angelica, Garlic (also pink ray), Jasmine (also pink ray)

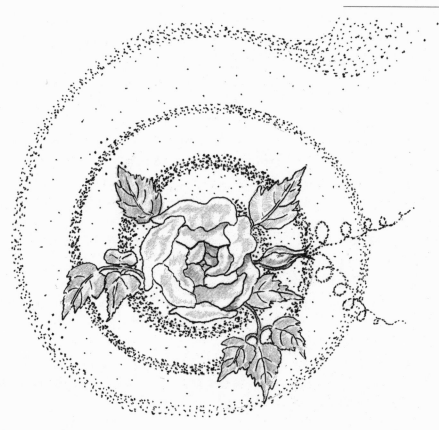

The Colours of Plants

HEALING GREEN

Green is nature's healing colour, and we naturally seek out a green place when we feel stressed or 'off colour'. It is no accident that the plant kingdom is this colour, for the green ray has specific healing power which is best suited to creating a healthy environment in which all life can flourish.

Everything in the universe is made up of the interplay of energy which is present in varying proportions in all living things. On a physical plane, life-force energy (prana or Ch'i), is differentiated into two opposite but complementary forces, Yin and Yang. Yang is the masculine force which has a positive electrical charge, is warm and active and represents light. Its colour is red, the colour of the blood which flows through our body giving us strength and vitality. Red also contains magnetic earth energy and has the effect of literally keeping our feet on the ground.

Yin is the feminine force which has a negative electrical charge, is cold and receptive in nature and represents darkness. Blue embodies Yin energy, and is the colour of oxygen, the oceans and the sky. This is the colour which lifts our spirits, helping us to connect to our intuition and higher self. Like magnets, the two polarities of red and blue, are opposing but complementary forces which attract each other.

Neither total lightness or total darkness represented by the colours red and blue-violet can support life, and it is only when a third binding force comes into action, that a stable environment is created. Cohesion is brought about through the colour green. Green is neutral and unifying and this is why the plant kingdom holds our atmosphere in balance so that life can exist on earth. The colour green is found in the centre of the visible spectrum is made up of equal amounts of Yin and Yang energy which gives it a perfect balancing and harmonising quality. The green vibration, has neither a short nor a long wavelength and it is neither hot

38

nor cold. This normalising action upon the earth promotes health and unity between all living things and in us, unity between our body, mind and spirit.

POLARITIES AND YIN/YANG ENERGY FOUND IN PLANTS AND MAN
Green is the harmonising force

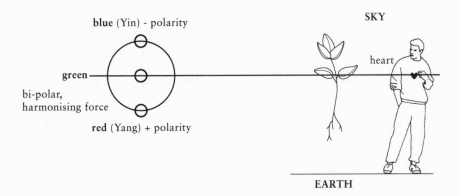

Although humankind is linked to the earth through our physical body, we are also linked to the sky through our subtle bodies. Like a pendulum, we swing constantly between the two polarities of red and blue; at one time attracted to the sensory world of the body while at other times rejecting our animal instincts and aspiring to our intuitive and spiritual connections.

We have to learn to reconcile the fact that we are of the body (red) and the spirit (blue) and in order to keep these two aspects of ourselves in balance we need the harmonising energy from the green ray. Green energy flows through our heart centre linking us through love to all nature and other people.

It is through universal love and our heart centre that we interconnect with all life for although plants and animals have very different physical form, at an energetic level we are surprisingly similar. Cells of plants and humankind are identical in all ways except for one – a magnesium molecule is found at the centre of chlorophyll, while iron is at the centre of haemoglobin. Iron is the core of haemoglobin, which is the basis of animal life and gives blood its red colouring. The basis of plant life is chlorophyll which gives it its characteristic green colouring and at the centre of the cell is magnesium.

**THE CELLS OF A PLANT AND ANIMAL ARE IDENTICAL EXCEPT
FOR THE CENTRAL MOLECULE**

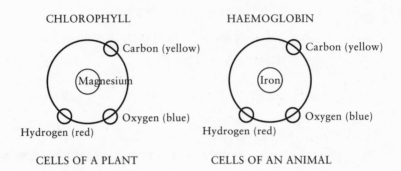

CELLS OF A PLANT   CELLS OF AN ANIMAL

While plants are dependent on sunlight, the animal kingdom is totally dependent on plants for its sustenance and well-being. Plants utilise the pure light energy from the sun and magnetic earth energy and change it into a form which can easily be utilised by the animal kingdom. All animals eat vegetables which contain chlorophyll, either directly or indirectly, and use it to build up red blood cells by creating haemoglobin. To do this, we have to transmute energy. In order to synthesise our own iron, our body changes the magnesium element in chlorophyll into iron by adding two atoms of oxygen, from the air we breathe.

Although plants give us physical nourishment to build up our red blood cells, they also provide us with blue vibrational energy. Chlorophyll absorbs light heavily in the red and blue range of the spectrum and as sunlight strikes the leaf, the green colouring of the plant reflects this merging of the two primal forces. Then a wonderful thing happens, the light-activated chlorophyll splits the water molecule, yielding a hydrogen atom. When this happens it also releases some oxygen (blue) into the air. We are then able to breathe in the oxygen and the blue energy into our body and these vibrations counter-balance the red energy within us.

FINDING BALANCE IN OUR LIVES

If we are to enjoy lasting good health we need to maintain a balance of colour energy in our system, but because we have red blood flowing through us we have a natural colour bias to the warm end of the spectrum. This is not difficult to recognise as we are warm-blooded creatures. If the red ray within us is left unchecked it keeps us bound up in our animal nature and the physical world and denies us access to the other more evolved parts of our being.

Imbalances occur when the flow of energy is blocked somewhere in our system with the result that there is a build up of the red ray within our system. If we have too much red, this will result in the quickening of our pulse and heart beat, a rise in blood pressure and temperature. Our face becomes flushed and we become impatient, irritable, aggressive and quick to temper. People who wish to control their environment or other people often have red energy suppressed somewhere in their chakra system.

When our system becomes disharmonious through a build-up of one colour vibration, we are naturally attracted to the opposite polarity. If we have too much Yang present this will result in a craving for Yin, so we would subconsciously be drawn to Yin colours, food, people and places which would soothe, calm and cool us.

If on the other hand we have too much blue (Yin) energy, we become cold and lethargic. Our blood pressure drops, our muscles sag, and we become depressed or weepy. If we are to find wholeness and peace we need to find balance by creating harmony between the red and blue energy within us.

Although Yang attracts Yin, just like two magnets, when they get too close they repel each other and the pendulum then starts to swing the other way. When we are in disharmony we constantly move between the extremes of yang and yin energy. The only way to stop the rocking motion is to utilise green energy embodied in nature. This provides us with the healing and balancing qualities required to keep both aspects of our psyche in harmony.

So nature has provided us with the elements of the three primary colour vibrations; green from plants, blue from oxygen and red from our blood. If we can maintain a flow of energy through our system, harmony can be maintained on all levels of our being. As the plant kingdom reflects this complete and balanced array of light energy, the next time we look at a humble plant we should give thanks and marvel at this wonder which gives us life.

THE 'ESSENCE' OF ESSENTIAL OILS

Not only has nature created the ideal atmosphere in which we can live, but also given us the tools for keeping us in perfect health.

Of all the life forms, plants catch the sunlight and through their own unique alchemy combine it with the energy from the earth to make the food which sustains all living things. Plants utilise sunlight for their life and growth, locking up the life-energy derived from the coloured cosmic rays. If properly preserved, this life-energy can have a powerful effect on us and one of the best ways of capturing the vibratory pattern of the light waves is by the preparation and use of essential oils.

Unlike other herbal preparations which are made up of plant material alone, essential oils contain the vibrational element which is the very 'essence' of the plant. Oil is used as the medium into which the essence of the plant is captured. Liquids are generally the most sensitive carriers of vibrations. This is shown by sound which travels much further under water than through the air and a stone dropped into a pond has a greater effect than dropping it in the ground. So preserving plant material in dry form results in it losing most of its vibrational quality which would have been preserved in the liquid essence.

Most oils are heavy and greasy substances, which remain unchanged when exposed to air. Essential oils, however, have a volatility which enables them to evaporate into the air and as they do so the scent develops. This is the spiritual nature of the essence. If you sniff an essential oil in the bottle its scent may be overpowering and even unpleasant, but as the oil evaporates the aroma takes on its true form. This metamorphosis from a visible oil into an invisible vibration allows essential oils to enter into the realm of the spiritual planes.

This vibrational pattern of essential oils has a very different mode of action compared with other plant preparations, with regard to how they interact with the human system. Unlike other types of herbal medicine, essential oils not only cause chemical changes to occur in the bloodstream, but have psycho-spiritual effects which respond to the colour and aroma vibrations held within them.

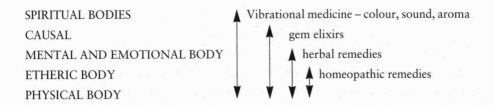

As colour and aroma is an integral part of an essential oil it makes it a wonderful medium for introducing healing vibrations into our system. The aroma molecules in essential oils enter our body through our skin, causing chemical reactions occur which bring about many physical, emotional and mental changes. On a vibrational level, different oils have affinities with different parts of the body which have a natural sympathetic resonance. Like colour, the aroma vibrations permeate our aura, and work on our etheric body through the chakra system and the network of energetic meridians. The vibrations of colours and aroma which are in tune with our inner energetic vibrations can have a significant effect on us, releasing blocked energy from our emotional body.

Since ancient times we have made medicines from plants knowing that plants contain this ethereal life-force energy. During this last century scientists have been able to reproduce the chemical make-up of plant cells in order to make drugs, but these artificially produced copies have been proven to be less effective in healing and many drug companies are now subsidising the growing of medicinal plants and trees.

As with the pharmacological effects of essential oils when they enter the bloodstream, water is an important transmitting medium when it comes to transference of the healing vibrational patterns. Water is the perfect transmitter of electro-magnetic vibrations, so by a method of transference the essence of the plant can be transferred to water without loss of its potency or qualities. It is interesting to know that even if some essential oil particles contact only a few molecules of water, there is a transference of the energy pattern or vibrational blueprint throughout the water.

This phenomenon is particularly useful for the colour aromatherapist, for the introduction of colour and aroma vibrations to any part of the body will result in the energetic vibrations being transferred to all cells with a sympathetic vibration through the water element flowing through our body.

Just as the quality of the food we eat affects our health and vitality, so the quality of the colour and aroma vibrations we direct into our system have an effect on their healing power. If the perfect vibratory pattern of the light waves is to be retained in the essential oil, it is vital that great care and attention is paid to the collection of the plant material, its preparation and the extraction process. The time of day, season, condition of the plant and conditions surrounding the extraction process will all influence the purity and potency of the vibrations carried by the essential oil.

Making an essential oil is similar to making a digital recording of your voice pattern onto a compact disc. In order to get a perfect recording you would have to make sure your energy levels were high and that you were in good health. As digital recordings are highly sensitive to sound vibrations, you would also have to make sure you made the recording at a place and time when there was no other noise or other vibrational interference. You would also need to make sure your recording equipment was appropriate, well maintained and clean and that you stored the disc safely at a temperature which would not affect its quality.

Unfortunately it is difficult to measure the quality of essential oils without chemical analysis, and even if this were to show you had a high quality oil, it would not necessarily reveal the vibrational potency of the oil. We can, however, use the price of the oil and the information provided by the supplier as a good indication of the purity of the essential oil.

It is better to develop our own judgement by using our own abilities to access an oil by its consistency, colour and aroma. By inhaling the aroma and gazing at the colour we can quickly develop our sensitivity to the therapeutic qualities of an oil and by using our sixth sense, we will know to what level of our subtle bodies the vibrations can penetrate. Some healers prefer to use a pendulum to check the quality of an oil.

The larger the arc drawn by the pendulum, the stronger the vibrations contained in the oil. We also need to check that the vibrations are of a positive kind, and this will be indicated by the direction of the swing. Each person needs to establish which direction the pendulum will move in, to show positive or negative energy. This direction will remain constant for each of us for all subsequent tests. By connecting to your higher mind the pendulum can reflect the potency and vibrational content of the oil.

FINDING COLOUR SIGNATURES

All plants reflect green energy, because in order to perform their life-giving function, they need to absorb sunlight. It is only in the presence of sunlight that plants unfold their leaves and through the presence of chlorophyll, which gives the plant its green colouring, are able to absorb and process light energy and finally store it in a form which can be easily absorbed by animals.

Plants change vital light energy into food through a process of transmutation. The German philosopher and scientist, Goethe, recognised this transformative property and described the green leaf as being the primal organ which linked the earth with the cosmic forces.

As the plant develops and aspires upwards towards the light, it converges into a point which holds the potential of all its future possibilities. As the bud develops, it loses its green colouring as it no longer serves the purpose of light-absorption. It is at this stage that the bud takes on the colour energy which will reveal its life-giving and healing qualities. Following in Goethe's footsteps, Rudolph Steiner also recognised the spiritual qualities of colour. He says 'Colour is the soul of Nature and the Cosmos, and we become aware of this soul when we experience colour.' As the flower opens to reveal its true colours, it will also develop and release a scent. These fine healing vibrations will permeate out from the plant and carried in the ether. It is only by tapping into the etheric that we are able to experience this spiritual energy.

The combined vibratory patterns of light and aroma create an energy-field around the plant which will attract pollination by insects, birds and animals. These creatures naturally perceive and react to the aura of the plant which they will utilise for food and natural healing. Being part of the animal kingdom, we also depend on plants for food, and can use plants to help keep us in good health. Unlike other creatures that live in harmony with plants, we have moved away from nature and as this separation increased, we have also lost our intuitive ability to read the patterns of colour and aroma in plants.

James Redfield suggests in his book *The Celestine Prophecy*, that in order to regain this ability, we first have to raise our awareness and appreciation of the beauty found in the natural kingdom. He says 'When we perceive something as beautiful it stands out from the background as more intense.' By heightening our awareness to colour and aroma and under-standing the messages they convey, we can heighten our sensitivity to the healing qualities of plants.

In order to discover which pattern of light energy the plant contains we can use the 'doctrine of signatures', which gives us information about the energy system of the plant as a whole and the impact and potency of individual parts. The shapes and colours of the roots, stems, leaves, flowers and seeds are personal markers or signatures which indicate the type of healing energy they contain.

When discovering the colour signature of essential oils we need to con-sider from which part of the plant the oil is derived. Some oils are made from the flowers, while other oils are made from the leaves, root, stems or seeds. The colours of these particular parts will give the plant its main colour signature. We should remember that the 'essence' flows through-out the whole eco-system of the plant so that every part reflects the healing qualities of this colour energy. So it may be that although the leaves were distilled to extract the essential oil, it will also contain some magnetic energy from the roots or electrical energy from the flowers. These are secondary healing colours which can be used to reinforce the action of the signature colour.

Some essential oils are made from roots, and although these will be predominantly Yang in nature, they will also hold the genetic vibration pattern for the whole plant. This is especially true if the plant propagates by runners, for the cells along the root will hold the blueprint which can create an entire new plant.

There are some plants that do not contain chlorophyll and cannot produce their own food. Like animals they must get their energy ultimately from green plants. Such plants do not need to live in light and may grow in soil or in other dark places. The simplest form is algae and the most complex are the fungi. These plants contain magnetic earth energy, rich in physical nutrients and minerals, which can influence our physical body and mind. Magic mushrooms have been used by many cultures to liberate the lower mind but because of their low vibrations they are not able to nourish our higher mind and spiritual bodies. The narcotic power of certain fungi and plant material lies in its ability to give us access to the cosmic consciousness by freeing us of the restriction of our physical senses.

The flower is the most evolved part of the plant containing the purest colour vibrations, and so its colour will indicate the light vibration which will have the ability to balance and heal the deepest levels of our being. Many flowers have colours which are not visible to the human eye. Golden-yellow flowers particularly have ultra-violet markings which attract bees and butterflies who are sensitive to these rays. Many yellow flowers contain this complementary violet energy.

Many essential oils are made from more than one part of the plant and it is not uncommon to find an oil derived from both leaves and flowers. In these cases the plant may hold more than one colour signature and there are some oils which contain several colour signatures.

As we know, colour energy is a vibration which can permeate our subtle bodies and energy system. Each colour vibration penetrates to different levels where healing is needed. When a plant has more than one colour signature, the different colour energy patterns released by the treatments will travel to different parts of our being. Each colour vibration acts upon different levels of our being. The secondary colour vibrations are useful as supportive colour treatments to reinforce the healing action of the main colour vibration.

Each essential oil has an affinity with a particular energy centre, and this is usually linked to the note and the Yin/Yang quality of the oil. Some Yang oils only permeate the lower bodies, and this makes them useful for treating physical ailments while other oils have a higher frequency which can permeate our subtle bodies, healing the emotions, mind and spiritual levels. Basil (*Ocimum basilicum*), which has a yellow colour signature, and high note (YIN) will nourish not only the solar-plexus but also the crown. Jasmine which has a white colour signature also contains red healing energy which will harmonise the base chakra with the crown.

The different colour vibrations work on different levels of our being through the chakras to which they relate. Essential oils made from roots and stem, act upon the lower three chakras and our physical body. This is why most oils made from the Yang parts of the plant also reflect magnetic colours of red, orange and gold. The colour of leaves indicates the healing colour which will balance the heart and the middle chakras, while the colour of the stem and roots indicates the healing colour relating to the lower chakras. As most leaves are green and many are heart shaped, essential oils made from leaves interact with the heart chakra and energy from the soul.

The parts which are exposed to sunlight for a longer period of time means that the energy becomes more refined and the light vibrations filled with vital colour energy and aroma. The flower is a celebration of this evolution and it bursts forth with light and perfume. Essential oil from flowers permeates our subtle bodies through the higher mind, while the perfume connects us to the spiritual realms.

As seeds mature, the light energy absorbed by them transforms from electrical to magnetic, for when the seed is released it needs nourishment of earth energy if it is to grow. Many fruits and seeds reflect this transformation of energy within them reflecting a deep indigo and violet colouring. Oils made from juniper berries, vanilla pods and clove reflect this mixture of Yin and Yang energy which contain both the red and blue ray.

The darker and more dense the colour of the plant, the more light energy is reflected away from the plant. These plants work upon the etheric and physical body. The paler and more translucent the plant, the more light energy it contains. Flowers with clear, iridescent colours are extremely powerful and work through the astral and mental bodies while softer, lighter versions of the same colour work on a higher level of consciousness and through the spiritual bodies.

Sometimes it is the colour of the oil itself which reflects a plant's true colour signature. It some cases certain vibrations are only released after extraction, giving the essential oil a surprising colouring. Often colour signatures revealed by this process of transformation, reveal the healing qualities of the plant on the subtle level which are linked to their life-quality (see section on life-qualities of colour page 6).

Yarrow is a good example of an oil made from pink flowers which becomes a deep indigo after processing. Yarrow is ruled by Venus with feminine nurturing qualities of the colour pink but in the physical body its therapeutic quality works on the bone marrow by stimulating blood renewal. The Indigo ray is the colour vibration associated with the skeletal system and particularly to the growth of bones.

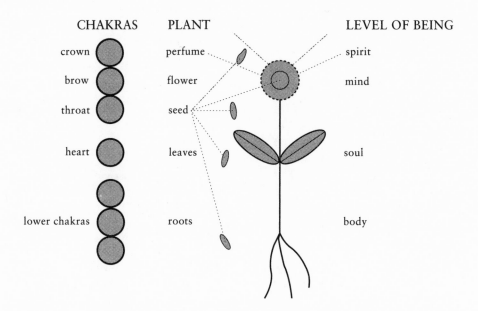

CHAKRAS	PLANT	LEVEL OF BEING
crown	perfume	spirit
brow	flower	mind
throat	seed	
heart	leaves	soul
lower chakras	roots	body

Nearly all plants are green in order for them to photosynthesise and live, so all medicine derived from plants has the harmonising and healing qualities of the colour green. So while all essential oils will contain some green energy, it is better to look at the colours of the flowers and stems when accessing the colour signature. Plants which do have a green signature colour category include some grasses, evergreen trees and green herbs. Many plants which have aromatic green leaves, have the green colour signature as it is the leaves, rather than the flowers which have the scent signature. Some plants have a green colour signature due to their shape, and many heart-shaped green leaves indicate a presence of healing green energy which opens and balances the heart chakra.

In order to find the main colour signature, aroma can be of assistance. If the flower is aromatic, then this vibration has the most pervasive effect. An aromatic leaf or root will make this the stronger vibration. If the flower, leaves and root are aromatic, then the colour signatures are of equal strength. The secondary healing colours related to the colours of the other parts of the plant will nourish the chakras to which they are related.

The main colour signature is, therefore, derived from the part of the plant from which the essential oil is made, while the colour and aroma of the oil indicates the note from which we can discover the level of healing for which the oil is particularly beneficial.

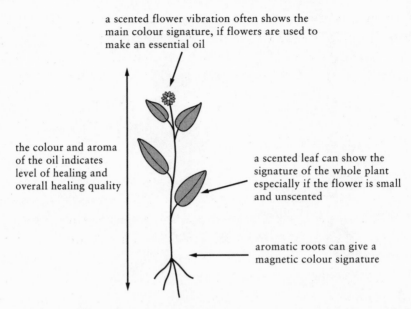

a scented flower vibration often shows the main colour signature, if flowers are used to make an essential oil

the colour and aroma of the oil indicates level of healing and overall healing quality

a scented leaf can show the signature of the whole plant especially if the flower is small and unscented

aromatic roots can give a magnetic colour signature

By combining Colour with aromatherapy we can draw upon the life force energy within the plant. The energy is not just of a general type but a specific one, each essential oil capturing a specific colour wavelength and vibrationary pattern.

Colour aromatherapy is still in its infancy, and is not a scientifically based therapy. It brings together a mixture between theory and proven experiments linking these with intuitive knowledge. There is much work to be done, and every student of colour aromatherapy can undertake their own research and development of the study, making a contribution to the progress and use of this branch of colour and aromatherapy. Not everyone will agree on the exact colour signatures. My analysis comes with tuning into the plant in its natural habitat where possible and using this sensitivity together with my knowledge and understanding of the action and healing qualities of each plant. We should strive to combine ancient wisdom, medical herbalism and shamanism with current research work in aromatherapy.

To avoid confusion, I have identified the one main colour signature of each oil and given a second or third minor signature if the oil acts on more than one level.

Sometimes it is difficult to decide on the exact colour signature of an oil and is most difficult when considering oils of a red, magenta or pink colour frequency. The quality of the oil itself can help us in these cases. Thick oils are more Yang and so relate to the longer wave-lengths of orange and red. Thinner, watery oils are more Yin and will contain lighter vibrations of pink. A rich, heavy or spicy perfume is sympathetic to lower frequencies while light, dry aromas will vibrate on higher frequencies. Highly penetrating, fresh herbaceous and bitter-sweet scents are usually connected with the middle colour vibrations of pale yellow and green. Magenta ray oils combine yang and yin qualities for although they have a deep colour signature, the aroma will be light.

Beautiful sweet or floral scents have low or high frequencies depending on the colour of the flowers from which the absolute is made. Rose oils particularly, can vary in colour signature depending on the origin and quality of the oil. Some types of Jasmine oil will have a red frequency due to the extraction process while another Jasmine oil will have lighter vibrations and be more in sympathy with magenta. For healing, it is better to use oils with an affinity to the pink colour ray in cases where red is contra-indicated or where the person is too weak to cope with the powerful effect of red.

In the Colour signature table at the end of this chapter I have given oils a red, pink and magenta classification according to the colour signature of the flowers only, although it would be wise to check the exact colour association of individual oils before use.

I find it helpful to make use of a pendulum in distinguishing between oils of similar types. Hold the pendulum above each bottle in turn, and ask whether the oil is red, magenta or pink. Make sure you know which way your pendulum will swing for a yes answer and a no answer before you begin. If you pendulum does not swing clearly in either direction, try again. If you still do not get a clear answer, it may be that the oil vibrates on both levels. The pendulum itself has no power, but is merely a tool which connects with the vibrations coming from your unconscious mind. This part of the mind has access to universal or cosmic consciousness. Everyone can draw on this universal pool of knowledge by tapping into their higher mind or 'intuition'.

The following table is helpful for discovering the colour signature of an essential oil at a glance. The overall healing colour of the plant may be different and you will need to look more fully at the signature of the whole plant in order to understand its overall healing quality. I have found that knowing the colour signature of the oil is useful when giving a combined colour-aroma treatment. The colour signature is helpful when selecting oils for blending, and secondary colours can be used in separate reinforcing colour treatments using lamps, gemstones, colour breathing and visualisations. The overall healing colour can also be introduced into the diet, dress and home environment of the person as this colour energy needs to be absorbed over a long period of time.

Note:

In reality the rainbow colours are not clearly separated but blend into each other. So there are a whole variety of tones between red and orange, orange and yellow, yellow and green and so on. Many essential oils have colour signatures which reflect colours which are not true rainbow hues but one of these half-tones. When this happens, the oil will reflect the qualities of the two rainbow colours between which they lie.

A RANGE OF COLOURS FALL BETWEEN RED, ORANGE AND YELLOW

◀──▶

RED, scarlet, orange-red, ORANGE, peach, apricot, gold, golden-yellow, YELLOW

Peach contains both orange and yellow energy, while scarlet is a mixture of red and orange. Yellow and green often work in harmony and many essential oils have yellow-green or green-yellow signatures. Oils such as parsley, petitgrain, lemon, basil and bergamot all have yellow and green energy in varying proportions. These oils combine the qualities of yellow and green, and differ from the healing actions of oils which may have a golden-yellow or dark green signature only. The main difference between the actions of Gold and yellow is that yellow works through the central nervous system and the lower mind, while Gold works through the higher mind and the subtle bodies.

In the following table, colours divided with a hyphen, for example pink – green, indicates that both colour signatures are present and should be used together. Colours divided by an oblique sign, for example red / orange, indicates a two colour signature due to more than one part of the plant being used. Red may reflect the colour signature where roots are used for extraction of the oil, while orange may reflect the colour signature if the stem is also used.

THE COLOUR SIGNATURES OF ESSENTIAL OILS

Plant name	Part used to make essential oil	Colour signature
ANGELICA (Angelica archangelica)	seeds, roots	white/pale yellow
ANISEED (Pimpinella anisum)	seeds	orange/gold
ANISE-STAR (Illicium verum)	fruit	green
BASIL (Ocimum basilicum)	flowering tops and leaves	leaves – yellow-green flowers – purple/white
BAY (Laurus nobilis)	leaf	green/indigo
WEST INDIAN BAY (Pimenta racemosa)	leaves	orange (indicated by colour of oil)
BENZOIN (Styrax benzoin)	gum	red/orange
BERGAMOT (Citrus bergamia)	peel	green/yellow
BIRCH (Betula – alleghaniensis, pendula, lenta)	bark/twigs	yellow/violet
BLACK PEPPER (Piper nigrum)	fruit	red
CAJUPUT (Melaleuca leucadendron)	leaves and twigs	yellow/violet
CAMPHOR (Cinnamomum camphora)	wood	red
CARAWAY (Carum carvi)	seeds	orange/gold/pink
CARDAMOM (Elettaria cardamomum)	seeds	orange/gold
CARROT SEED (Daucus carota)	seeds	yellow-orange/violet
CEDARWOOD (Juniperus virginiana) (Cedrus atlantica)	wood	red/orange/yellow
CELERY (Apium graveolens)	seeds	yellow/green/orange

Plant name	Part used to make essential oil	Colour signature
CHAMOMILE (Anthemis nobilis) – Roman (Matricaria chamomilla) – German	dried flowers	white/deep-blue (German) white/blue (Roman) (indicated by colour of oil)
CINNAMON (Cinnamomum zeylanicum)	bud, bark, leaf	orange/indigo
CITRONELLA (Cymbopogon nardus)	leaf (grass)	yellow
CLARY SAGE (Salvia sclarea)	Flowering tops and leaves	magenta/violet a mixture of white – blue – red
CLOVE (Eugenia caryophyllata)	dried bud	indigo which contains red energy
CORIANDER (Coriandrum sativum)	seeds	yellow/green/pink
CUMIN (Cuminum cyminum)	fruit (seeds)	yellow also contains pink energy
CYPRESS (Cupressus sempervirens)	cones and leaves	blue/orange
DILL (Anethum graveolens)	fruit	yellow
EUCALYPTUS (Eucalyptus globulus)	leaves	green/pink (some varieties blue)
FENNEL (Foeniculum vulgare)	seeds	yellow
FIR (Abies balsamea)	needles and leaves	green
FRANKINCENSE (Boswellia carteri)	bark	violet
GARLIC (Allium sativum)	stems and pods	pink/white
GERANIUM (Pelargonium graveolens/ odorantissimum)	flowers and leaves	pink/green
GINGER (Zingiber officinale)	root	orange/yellow/blue
GRAPEFRUIT (Citrus paradisi)	peel	yellow/violet

Plant name	Part used to make essential oil	Colour signature
HYSSOP (*Hyssopus officinalis*)	leaves and flowering tops	blue/violet
JASMINE (*Jasminum grandiflorum*)	flowers	white/red/deep pink (revealed in colour of oil)
JUNIPER (*Juniperus communis*)	berries	indigo
LAVENDER (*Lavendula officinalis*)	flowers	violet blue (Spike Lavender)
LEMON (*Citrus limonum*)	peel	yellow/green
LEMONGRASS (*Cymbopogon citratus*)	leaves	yellow
LIME (*Citrus medica*)	peel	green
LINDEN BLOSSOM (*Tilia europaea*)	flowers	yellow (relates to the honey nectar in the flowers)
MANDARIN (*Citrus madurensis*)	peel	orange/blue
MARJORAM (*Origanum marjorana*)	leaves and flowering heads	blue/orange
MARIGOLD (*Calendula officinalis*)	flowers	yellow/green
MELISSA (*Melissa officinalis*)	leaves and flowers	pink – green
MYRRH (*Commiphora myrrha*)	stem and branches	red/deep pink (related to the gum resin)
MYRTLE (*Myrtus communis*)	leaves	blue – green (Turquoise) indigo
NEROLI (*Citrus aurantium*)	petals	orange/yellow (colour of the oil)
NIAOULI (*Melaleuca viridiflora*)	leaves and shoots	turquoise, yellow/purple (from flowering tips)
NUTMEG (*Myristica fragrans*)	seeds	orange
ORANGE (*Citrus vulgaris*)	peel	orange

Plant name	Part used to make essential oil	Colour signature
ORIGANUM (Origanum vulgare)	leaves and flowering tops	green – purple/yellow
PALMAROSA (Cymbopogon martini)	leaves	green
PARSLEY (Petroselinum sativum)	seed	green/yellow (revealed in the colour of the oil)
PATCHOULI (Pogostemon patchouli)	leaves	red/violet and orange (revealed in the colour of the oil)
PEPPERMINT (Mentha piperita)	leaves and flowering tops	green/violet
PETITGRAIN (Citrus vulgaris)	leaves and young shoots	green/pale yellow
PIMENTO (Pimenta officinalis)	leaf and fruit or berry	orange/indigo (revealed in the blue-black shell of the fruit)
PINE (Pinus sylvestris)	needles and cones	blue/orange
ROSE (Rosa centifolia) Cabbage Rose	petals	red/deep pink
ROSE (Rosa damascena) Damask Rose	petals	pink – peach/green
ROSE (Rosa gallica) Red Rose	petals	red
ROSEMARY (Rosmarinus officinalis)	flowers	blue
ROSEWOOD (Aniba rosaeaodora)	heartwood	pink
SAGE (Salvia officinalis), (Salvia lavandulaefolia) (Spanish)	leaves	violet/blue
SANDALWOOD (Santalum album)	roots and heartwood	violet/yellow
STAR ANISE – Illicium verum	fruits	green

Plant name	Part used to make essential oil	Colour signature
THYME (Red) (*Thymus vulgaris*)	leaves and flowers	red/green
TEA – TREE (*Melaleuca alternifolia*)	leaves	indigo/yellow
VERBENA (*Lippia citriodora*)	stalks and leaves	green – pink
VETIVERT (*Andropogon muricatus*)	root	yellow
VIOLET (*Viola odorata*)	leaves and flowers	green and violet
YARROW (*Achillea millefolium*)	flowers	indigo/pink (revealed in the oil)
YLANG – YLANG (*Cananga odorata*)	flowers	magenta – deep pink/yellow

SPIRITUAL MESSAGES OF PLANTS

Not only does nature provide us with healing for the body, it also gives us tools to heal the mind and spirit. So while plants provide us with food and medicine to keep our physical body in good health, we can also absorb their fragrance and colour energy within them to uplift, inspire, satisfy and revitalise our subtle bodies.

Illness is a reflection of disharmony in our subtle bodies but no real healing can take place without a shift in consciousness in every part of our being. Illness brings with it a message of the need for change, and unless there is movement of energy within our conscious and unconscious being we can never eliminate the real cause of disharmony.

Essential oils work on all the levels of our being simultaneously, flooding our aura with balancing and healing vibrations. This effect is largely unconscious and we are often only aware of the harmonious changes within us when we experience a state of well-being. Oils also contain secondary healing colours related to the colours of the other parts of the plant and these will nourish the chakras to which they are related.

Vibrational energy is able to disperse stagnant energy, restoring vitality to the chakras, and charging the aura with protective vibrations. If healing is to be permanent we also need to consciously adjust the vibrations in our mental and emotional bodies.

While many people are quite happy to make use of herbal and vibrational plant preparations, we have been more reluctant to make use of the healing prescriptions they carry for conscious self-healing.

The messages which the colour and aroma carry relate to challenges and lessons we have to learn in order for our soul to evolve and grow. This transformation is ensures healing at a spiritual level. Dr Christine Page, a leading light in complementary healing, says that our journey on earth is to work towards union of the physical and spiritual aspects within us. She says 'the purpose of life is to increase the level of consciousness through the interaction between spirit and matter until ultimately there is no separation between these two aspects of polarity and the consciousness of the soul and the source become one.'

The life-quality and lesson each plant has for us, links to a healing colour which it reflects on this subtle level. In order to discover the life-quality and lesson the plant has to teach us we need to look at each plant as a total living system which includes the climate and location where it grows, its relation to other plants and natural elements as well as its shape, colour and aroma. (Refer to the table giving the colour, life-qualities and lessons on page 8) We can use the doctrine of signatures to find the life-quality and lesson the plant carries, but the personal challenge the plant carries for us only becomes clear through meditation while inhaling the aroma and colour of the flower or oil.

MIXING ESSENTIAL OILS USING COLOUR AS YOUR KEY

Using colour as the basis for mixing essential oil produces beautiful vibrational harmonies and is a simple way of creating oil blends for massage, bathing, or to burn in room diffusers.

Although we can use an individual aroma or colour for healing, often we need a several energetic vibrations to balance the body, mind and spirit. In order to create a colour-aroma harmony, we have to combine different notes on the colour scale similar to forming a chord or harmonic in music. We can do this by creating a harmony of colour by blending aromatic oils that have an affinity with those wavelengths. One way which is used by aromatherapists and perfumers to blend oils is by dividing them into plant family groups:

Woody *(Pinaceae)* – **Herbaceous** *(Labiatae)* – **Citrus** *(Rutceae)* – **Floral** *(Rosaceae)* – **Resinous** *(Busseraceae)* – **Spicy** *(Zingiberaceae)*

Each oil blends well with other oils in its group and with oils in the closest neighbouring group.

When we want to obtain a good mix of aroma and colour vibrations we can use the same principle, using colour to represent the qualities of each group. Essential oils can be divided into groups related to the following colours.

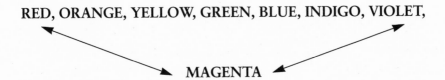

RED, ORANGE, YELLOW, GREEN, BLUE, INDIGO, VIOLET,

MAGENTA

A good blend can be obtained by mixing two oils of the same colour. So that two orange oils mix well together and so do two green oils. The second way of mixing oils using colour is by mixing colours with those of the neighbouring frequencies. Orange can be mixed with red or yellow, while indigo, blue or violet create a colour harmony. For red or violet oils this means the two colour frequencies to the right or left respectively.

If you wish to blend three oils, you can mix two blue with one violet, or two yellow with one orange. There are many permutations depending on the healing qualities you wish to convey. A chord of colour harmony can be achieved by mixing one oil from the bottom, one from the middle and one from the top notes – that is an oil from the long, middle and short colour frequency. This blend is excellent for balancing all the chakras.

(red, orange)	(yellow, green)	(blue, violet, magenta)
LONG	MIDDLE	SHORT
FREQUENCY	FREQUENCY	FREQUENCY
	WHITE	
	(all frequencies)	

It is usual for an essential oil to have resonance with a colour depending on its Yin or Yang quality, but it will also attract and have sympathy with the opposite and complementary colour.

So you can make an oil blend with a good mix of energy by mixing two complementary colours. The light waves of these oils when working synergistically, create the essence of white light. Complementary colours are wave-lengths of colour which are naturally attracted to each other. When one colour is present it pulls in its partner just as two magnets are pulled together by their opposite electrical polarity. Working with nature in this way we can create balanced blends using complementary colours. Mix a blend containing equal proportions of complementary colours.

COMPLEMENTARY COLOUR BLENDS

RED	is complementary to BLUE
MAGENTA/PINK	is complementary to GREEN
ORANGE	is complementary to INDIGO
YELLOW	is complementary to VIOLET
WHITE	harmonises green although it has no complementary

An harmonious red and blue blend could be made from Chamomile (blue) and Jasmine (red), or Chamomile (blue) and Ylang Ylang (red) or Rose (red). A yellow and violet complementary blend is Linden Blossom (yellow) and Lavender (violet) or Citronella (yellow) and Violet (violet). Geranium and Clary Sage would make a balanced green and magenta blend, while Orange (orange) and Juniper (indigo) mix well together.

You can also introduce complementary colour energy into a single oil if you energise the base oil under a coloured filter which instils it with that particular colour vibration. You can also solarise the oil blend with the sympathetic colour vibration by placing it under a coloured glass pyramid or filter or use healing colour treatments to reinforce the therapeutic action of the oil blends. (These methods are explained in chapter 5)

Here are some examples of ways to mix harmonious blends.

- Red oils mix well together
- Red oils mix well with orange and yellow (two neighbouring colours in the colour spectrum)
- Red oils mix well with their complementary colour green

- Blue oils mix well together
- Blue oils mix with green and violet (groups on either side of the colour spectrum)
- Blue oils mix well with their complementary colour orange

Oils which vibrate on the green ray, have a special place when creating a blend. The balancing and harmonising qualities of green allows this vibration to mix readily with almost all other colours. For this reason, beautiful green Geranium oil can be added successfully to most blends.

You can administer the colour healing before, or during an aromatherapy treatment, or, if the oil blend is to be used in the bath or room diffuser, colour can be introduced through colour breathing, colour lamps or candles.

COLOUR NOTES

Just as different oils have an affinity with a particular colour, two oils with the same colour may have different healing purposes depending on the amount of white light contained within that vibration. If we compare colours to musical notes, we know that there are several A and several C notes within audible range. Although all A notes will have the same harmonic, they will have different pitches depending whether they are a high A or a low A. So while Benzoin and Jasmine share a red colour signature, Benzoin oil will have a denser red vibration, or lower note, than Jasmine which is full of light energy and has a lighter vibration and high note. Many yellow oils have a top note because of the presence of the complementary colour, violet, which is found in the form of invisible ultra-violet markings on the flower.

If you are a qualified aromatherapist you may already blend essential oils through the process of 'notes' commonly used in perfumery. This is a means of dividing fragrances into TOP notes, MIDDLE notes and BASE notes. The base notes include aromas such as patchouli, jasmine and myrrh. Middle notes include geranium, lavender and marjoram, while top notes include such oils as eucalyptus, lemon and basil. Top notes are usually found in an oil made from the flower or leafy part of the plant rather than the stem, roots or seeds which are more Yang in nature. Top notes can also be found in some middle and a few base note oils where there is a balance of energy both from sunlight and the earth.

When comparing these notes to colour frequencies we can say that the:

BASE NOTES	red and orange,	rich and heavy scent (Yang energy)
MIDDLE NOTES	yellow and green	fragrance takes time to emerge
TOP NOTES	blue and violet	light quality due to fast evaporation (Yin)

Oils of the same colour frequency mix well together, so that a good top notes blue energy blend could be Yarrow, Juniper and Rosemary. A base note blend could include Sandalwood (orange), Black Pepper (red), Benzoin (red), Jasmine (red), or Rose (red).

Notes are helpful to pinpoint the healing range of an oil and to differentiate between the actions of oils with similar colour signatures. So although most red oils have a base note there are a few red oils with a middle or top note. Rose (Damask) has a red colour signature, but because it contains light energy locked into the petals, it has a top to middle note. White light resonates with the top notes of blue and violet, so oils with a corresponding colour signature such as myrrh, lavender and chamomile have top notes. Often oils with a pink colour vibration will have an affinity with green energy, giving an oil with a pink colour signature a middle note.

BASE NOTES	healing to the lower three chakras – physical and etheric bodies
MIDDLE NOTES	healing to the solar-plexus and heart chakras – astral and mental body

TOP NOTES   healing to the top chakras – spiritual bodies
MIXTURE OF BASE   balances the base and crown chakra – whole
AND TOP NOTES   aura

The therapeutic qualities of an essential oil are revealed by its colour signature and its note indicates the level of its action. Sandalwood is both a sedative and a tonic, so although it has an affinity with blue it also has an affinity with orange and a base note. The tonic action works on the nervous system while the sedative works on the mind. Cypress has a balancing green colour signature although it has a base note corresponding to the grounding energy in the oil. So the colour signature of the oil gives it healing qualities, while the note indicates its healing potential. Rose (centifolia) has a red-orange colour signature while having a top note. This indicates that while it promotes physical love, its vibrations pervade the spiritual bodies opening the soul to divine love.

Here is a selection of oils showing the colour affinity and note. The colour signature will indicate the chakra which is energised by the oil, while the note will show the energy centres which will also be affected.

Essential oil	Colour	Note	Promotes flow of energy between:
Basil	yellow/green	top	solar-plexus, heart, crown
Bergamot	yellow/green	top	solar-plexus, heart, crown
Black Pepper	red	base	base
Cardamom	orange	middle	sacral, solar-plexus
Cedarwood	red	top	base and crown
Chamomile	blue	top	throat, brow and crown
Cypress	green	base	base and heart
Clary Sage	deep pink	middle	heart
Geranium	pink/green	middle	heart
Fennel	yellow	top	solar-plexus and crown

Essential oil	Colour	Note	Promotes flow of energy between:
Frankincense	violet/gold	base	base, crown
Hyssop	blue/violet	middle	heart and brow, crown
Jasmine	red	middle	base and solar-plexus
Lavender	violet	top	crown
Marjoram	green	middle	heart
Melissa	yellow/green	middle/top	solar-plexus, heart, crown
Orange	orange	top	sacral and throat
Peppermint	green/violet	top	heart and crown
Patchouli	orange	base	base and sacral
Neroli	orange/yellow	middle/base	sacral and solar-plexus
Rose (centifolia)	red	top	base and crown
Rosemary	blue	middle/top	solar-plexus and brow
Sandalwood	orange	base	base and sacral
Ylang-Ylang	deep pink	middle	base and heart

Use the following list to help you mix harmonious essential oil blends. I have selected the most commonly used essential oils and listed the colour frequency related to the oils' affect on our emotional, mental and spiritual bodies.

QUICK COLOUR GUIDE FOR MIXING ESSENTIAL OILS

RED RAY OILS (complementary healing colour green)

Aphrodisiac/energising/grounding/toning/stimulating/motivating/aphrodisiac

Black Pepper	warming, penetrating, comfort and security, endurance
Cedarwood	power, strength, grounding, dignity, fortitude
Jasmine	apathy, rigidity of mind, secretive, restores self-confidence, shyness, harmonising, awareness

Benzoin	loneliness, sadness, warming and soothing, stimulates healing process
Sage	tiredness, depression, grief, quickens senses, wisdom, tonic for kidneys and liver
Camphor (White)	stimulating but balancing, cold, stiffness, rheumatics, nervousness
Myrrh	warming, heating, stimulates physical body to heal by building up strength
Rose (Red)	narcotic, aphrodisiac, linked to physical love, creativity and conception

PINK RAY OILS (complementary healing colour green)

These are gently stimulating to the physical body but act more on the emotions than red oils. Muscle relaxant, links to the feminine principle, nurturing and self-love.

Rose	passion, comforting PMT, sexual problems, soothing, grief, appreciation of love and beauty
Rosewood	soothing, relaxing, good for mood swings, stability
Palmarosa	water balance, aids cell regeneration, uplifts emotions
Melissa	humility, nurturing the female aspect, for over-sensitive states
Garlic	regulating thyroid, tonic, strengthens and detoxifies, uplifting

ORANGE RAY OILS (complementary healing colour blue)

Emotionally releasing, immune tonic, toning, improving self-esteem and a good self-image through appreciation of the physical form, clearing emotional baggage

Aniseed	invigorates the mind, builds self-esteem, frees emotions

Caraway	learning from past mistakes, wisdom, general tonic
Ginger	self-awareness, self-acceptance
Carrot Seed	tonic to reproductive system, relief from stress, clears bowels, cleansing effect on the mind, kidney stones
Bergamot	good for depression, anxiety, obsession, regret, lack of confidence, stress, shyness, negative thoughts, joy, uplifting
Pine	tired mind, eases breathing, stimulates circulation, muscular pain
Mandarin	skin toner, relentlessness, nervous tension during pregnancy, children's nervousness, digestive problems
Neroli	(also lifts sorrow, stress relief, nervous tension, mental strain, shock, yellow ray) fright, hysteria, disorientation, relentlessness
Nutmeg	anti-depressive, lifts mind, warming and sensual
Orange	tonic, joy, generosity, warmth, sharing
Patchouli	pervasive, clarity, decisive, expansion, clear thinking
Pimento	healing for shock, sharing, communication, insight
Sandalwood	intuition, worry about the future, over-sensitive, insecurity, (blue) encourages humility, cynicism, recurring dreams

YELLOW RAY OILS (complementary healing colour violet)

Mentally uplifting, feeds the nerves, memory and mental stimulant, warming without heat, mentally expanding, regaining personal power

Bergamot	soothing, healing, uplifting to mind and emotions, sedating
Birch	pain relief, dignity, purifying, transforming, balancing
Cardamom	clarifying, encouraging, enthusiasm, expansion, courage, fortitude, selfishness
Celery	tonic, sedative, discrimination, lightness, softness, strength

Coriander	stimulates circulation, aids memory, confidence, optimism, enthusiasm
Cajeput	warming and quickens pulse, penetrating, cynicism, improves memory, procrastination, compulsive habits i.e. eating disorders
Citronella	tonic, stomachic, insect repellent, deodorant
Cumin	free, communicative, warming, releasing, stimulating
Lemon	purifying, refreshing, sluggish, selfish, lacking motivation
Lemongrass	boredom, lack of interest, sulkiness, nervous exhaustion
Marigold	comforts the heart and spirits, anti-inflammatory, antiseptic
Grapefruit	releasing negative emotions like envy and jealousy, frustration, bitterness about the past, despondency, procrastination
Basil	clearing, poor memory, listless, lack of discipline, tired mind, lack of concentration, clarifying, awakening
Fennel	normalising, for strength, courage and longevity
Vetivert	debility, depression, nervous tension, muscular aches
Cinnamon	normalise liver function, energises the mind when mentally exhausted, gives direction
Camphor (Yellow)	cold compresses for bruises and sprains, calms digestion, constipation, good for nervous system when inhaled. Avoid taking Camphor oil internally
Sandalwood	insecurity, worry about future, over-sensitivity

GREEN (green complements any other colour as it acts as the balancing agent)

Balance, regulating circulation, healing the emotions, relaxing to the mind, expanding soul growth through a trust in the process of nature.

Cypress	calming action for talkative and irritable people, protection, wise, finding purpose through stillness, inner peace
Eucalyptus	cools emotions, clears mind, aids concentration, strengthens nerves
Geranium	harmonising, general healing and balance, stress, liver tonic, addictions
Fir	heals heart from shock, grief, feeling trapped, tired mind
Lime	sedative, tonic, carminative, migraine, headaches, insomnia, nervous tension and stress-related conditions
Linden Blossom	relaxing, calming, balanced, promotes sleep, normalises blood pressure, nervous tension
Peppermint	cooling, mentally stimulating, aids study, headache, nausea
Petitgrain	anxiety, depression, tranquilliser
Origanum	releases anxiety, anger, hysteria, stress
Parsley	cleansing emotions, clears head, gives space to breathe
Star Anise	aids digestion, carminative, relieves nausea, warming to respiratory system, PMT, encourages oestrogen production
Thyme Red	relieve nasal congestion, sore throat, chills, colds, stress related Influenza and Viral Infections
Verbena	soothing effect on parasympathetic nervous system, relaxing, refreshing

BLUE (complementary colour energy Orange)

Sedative, contracting in action, calming to the mind, aids self-expression, cooling of heat, inhibiting, linking to the intuition

German Chamomile	nerve sedative, relaxing, peace and patience, anxiety, tension, anger and fear

Roman Chamomile	generally soothing, restless mind, worry, tantrums, impulsiveness, hyperactive
Myrtle	soothing, cleansing emotions and mind
Marjoram	overwork, mental strain, hostility, irrational thoughts, warms and comforts, anxiety, sedative, loneliness and grief
Thyme (White)	bacterial for throat infections, antiseptic, strengthens nerves, activates brain cells aids memory, concentration, exhaustion, mental blocks and traumas
Rosemary	restorative, centring, clarity of vision, clear-sightedness, protection, mental strain, aids memory, hypotension, nervous complaints, psychic protection
Hyssop	focuses the mind, releases emotional pain through understanding, helps clear lungs, helps form scars and disperse bruising

INDIGO (complementary colour White)

Intuition, purification, rejuvenation, hypnotic, sedative, deep pain healer, develops inner vision.

Bay Laurel	warming to emotions, mildly narcotic, digestion, tonic by purifying action on reproductive system
Clove	strengthens memory, lifts depression, body/mind balance, antiseptic, pain relieving, respiratory aid
Tea-tree	antibiotic, purifier, toxin cleanser, antibacterial, antifungal
Yarrow	astringent, inflammations, circulation, acts on bone marrow, nervous tension, varicose veins, scars, wounds

VIOLET RAY OILS (complementary colour Yellow)

Purifying, antiseptic, stimulating without heat, transformative, protection against psychic forces, balancing the body, mind and spirit.

Juniper	blood purifying and cleansing, lethargy, protection, toxic elimination
Lavender	soothes immune system, balancing, anxiety, exhaustion, hysteria, hyperactivity, impatience, insomnia, insecurity, mood swings, negative thoughts
Frankincense	meditation, elevating, wisdom, rejuvenating, protection
Niaouli	firms tissues, aids healing, tissue stimulant, reviving and refreshing to the mind, helps communication
Spanish Sage	insomnia, headaches, nervous exhaustion, comforts the heart, sedative, longevity, protection against illness, banishes feelings of anxiety and anger
Violet	pain-relief, cleansing, mildly stimulating, sedates the conscious mind
Sandalwood	encourages humilty, intuition, prevents recurring dreams

MAGENTA (complementary colour green)

Emotionally warming and uplifting, caring and nurturing, balances the emotions, gently stimulating, renews vitality and life-force

| *Ylang Ylang* | confidence, sensual, emotionally soothing, euphoric, calms anger, guilt, impatience, panic, selfishness, stubbornness, suspiciousness, instils confidence. |
| *Clary Sage* | obsession, insomnia, overwork, PMT, panic, nerves, post natal depression, instils feeling of well-being, communication with the unconscious mind |

WHITE (all colours) – use with green for balance and to open the heart)

Enlightenment, encompassing, liberating, peace, spiritual release, purifying

| *Carnation* | stillness, originality, liberating, connectedness, tenderness |

Narcissus	hypnotic, mesmerising, meditative, vision, truth
Gardenia	seeing perfection and beauty, divine love
Angelica	opens spiritual channel from crown to base
Jasmine	inspiration, uplifting, raises physical love to spiritual love

———————

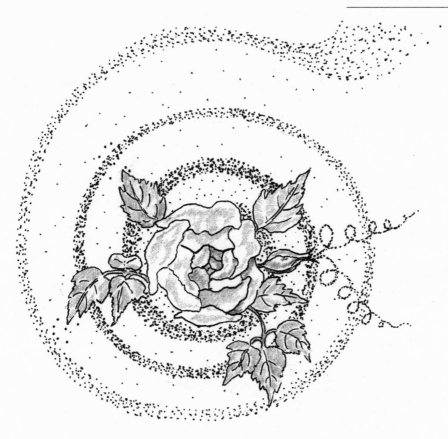

Colour and Aroma Treatments

SYNERGY OF COLOUR AND AROMA

Colour therapy and Aromatherapy work together to heal through a process of synergy. By introducing a harmonious mixture of aroma and colour vibrations into our energetic system, a healing effect is created which is far more potent than could be achieved by using either one or the other therapy.

Cooking a colourful and aromatic meal is a perfect example of this principle. It is the way the colours of the ingredients and aromatic flavouring react and blend with each other that creates the appetising and tasty end result. The proportions of the colours and aromas contribute to the success of the overall blend. The secret is in the blending so that the individual elements work harmoniously together. When you fail to do this you are creating 'bad synergy' which extends into the psychological and emotional factors causing an energy imbalance and thus ill health.

Most of us have experienced this synergy of colour and aroma ourselves when we have walked in a garden at sunset. It is at twilight that colour and perfume are drawn together out of the haze. Shape and form disappear into the darkness as the more spiritual qualities of flowers are highlighted. At dusk the air is charged with positive ions making it a time of stillness and contemplation when our senses become heightened and our sensitivity to subtle vibrations increased. As night approaches light coloured flowers take on a special translucency, while some only reveal their glory and perfume in moonlight. Often the evening is the time when sweet heady aromas of white jasmine, lilies or datura (moonflowers) pervade the atmosphere filling us with the feelings of sensuality, and love. The healing and spiritual vibrations emitted by white flowers can also best be appreciated after sunset and walking in a specially created 'moon' garden can inspire us with the feeling of purity, peace and grace.

Unfortunately we cannot always experience gardens by moonlight and we have to take in healing aromatic and colour vibrations in other ways. If we are to reap the benefits from the healing vibrations we need to be receptive to them. It is important, therefore, that we should spend time relaxing our mind and heightening our awareness to the subtle atmosphere before we begin any of the following treatments.

HEALING LAMPS

In order for us to be healthy we require a balance of colour energy contained within natural sunlight. Often, this natural energy balance becomes distorted by external factors such as pollution in our environment or by internal ones such as our emotional and mental state. When this imbalance occurs we need to introduce specific colour vibrations so that harmony is restored. As each energy centre in our etheric body has a natural sympathetic resonance with a colour wave-length, we can introduce individual colours to energise and nourish particular problem areas.

It is not always possible to use natural sunlight for healing, but it is possible to introduce healing colour vibrations into the human body, by artificial light. This is the basis of Colour Therapy. Coloured light can be used to flood the whole aura, and this type of overall diffused light therapy is known as Light Irradiation. This should not be confused with irradiation given to foodstuffs to make them last longer as this process involves bombarding food with ultra-violet light which kills the life-force energy.

Another fast developing area of light therapy is Chromotherapy. Rather than flooding the entire body with light, Chromotherapy involves the use of directional light, focused onto a specific organ, gland or area of the body. This method of using light to heal includes Colour reflexology and Colour acupuncture where a concentrated light beam is focused onto a particular chakra or receptive energy point on one of the meridians or foot reflexes.

When using an artificial light source it is usually focused through a colour filter made from acetate or coloured glass. This has the effect of cutting out all colour vibrations except the one which is the same colour as the filter. This colour wave-length passes through the filter and is absorbed into our physical and subtle bodies. Shining a light through a photographic acetate filter allows us to measure the exact colour and wave length administered enabling us to keep an accurate record of the effects of the colour energy. This method of applying light energy is favoured by those with a modern scientific approach to Colour Therapy.

In order to give light irradiation or Chromotherapy, you will need a selection of colour filters and a light source which can project light in a small area no bigger than a metre in diameter. Small spotlights, like those used in theatres or for shop displays, have been found to work well. One can also obtain coloured spotlight bulbs which you can fit into a regular table or standard lamp or overhead spots. These lights give off a good deal of heat and are quite bright so you need to use them with care and never directly in the eyes. They are, however, very useful for bouncing coloured light off a white wall or ceiling during an aromatherapy treatment. You can also shine them directly onto the back or the feet while a person is sitting or lying down.

The most popular way therapists introduce colour into a healing treatment is with the use of a Colour crystal torch. This torch is specially designed to project a fine beam of light through a coloured glass filter and clear quartz crystal. The crystal has the capacity to direct and amplify the light beam, turning a weak torch beam into a powerful healing tool. There are various healers working in light research, who have produced their own man-made crystal tips for sharp focus of the coloured beam used in these torches. The colour pulse torch is a similar torch which has a pulse facility, in order to create a rhythm of light vibration which is able to move and change energy patterns. There are several advantages to using torches to give colour healing. They are portable, and can be used to focus light on a foot reflex or meridian point as well as working on the chakras and energy in the aura as a whole.

Some practitioners prefer to use a light instrument to activate the foot reflexes and acupuncture points. The most widely used colour reflexology instrument is the 'Colour reflexology torch' which can be purchased from Colour Therapy suppliers. It consists of a Krypton torch with a fixed focus beam which is directed through a natural quartz crystal point which is hand selected for its magnifying properties. The cuff connecting the crystal to the torch head is made of copper, a metal chosen for its electro-magnetic conductive properties. The units available usually include a set of stained glass discs through which the light beam is directed onto the reflex point requiring treatment. The torch is held over the point for one to two minutes, or the pulse mechanism used whereby a pulsing colour vibration is set up.

When you wish to use the torch in pulse mode, the beam should be switched on for three seconds and turned off for two seconds. This should be continued for thirty seconds, the colour being projected six times in a thirty second period or twelve times over a minute.

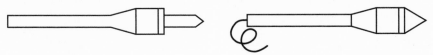

A. reflexology and colour acupuncture torch   B. pyramid focus manmade torch

In Germany, Peter Mandel, who practises Colour Acupuncture, has developed a purpose built electro-magnetic colour torch with a manmade pyramid point. This instrument can only be used in the controlled medical environment by practitioners specifically trained in its use. In Holland, a colour instrument which sends a pinpoint of light through a coloured gel is already in use.

If you do not wish to buy a reflexology torch, a cheaper and effective option is to use a clear quartz crystal point on the reflex, sending colour in the same way as you would by directing colour energy through your hands. When using a crystal rather than your fingers, you do not make physical contact with the feet nor do you exert pressure on the reflex. Hold the crystal so that it is just touching the reflex point and direct colour energy through your aura and the crystal. Clear quartz crystals are pyro-electric, absorbing and transmitting electrical impulses. When energy is directed into the crystal, it is transmitted to the other end, where the point intensifies the vibration before transmitting the impulse.

It is also possible to combine the quartz crystal treatment with essential oils or flower essences. Place a drop of an appropriate essential oil or flower essence on the tip of the crystal or torch before stimulating the reflex. The combined vibrations of the reflexology, colour and flower essence will have a 'synergistic' effect. You can also instil colour aroma vibrations into the reflexes and meridians by moving the crystal tip in spiralling movements above the points. Move the crystal in a downwards and clockwise movement to instil energy, and in an anti-clockwise and outward movement to draw out pain and negative energy.

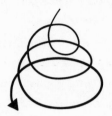

moving energy out - anti-clockwise

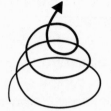

moving energy in - clockwise

Larger light instruments

It is also possible to send colour energy through whole areas of the body, the chakras, and the entire sole of the foot using light instruments in the same way as you do using the palms of your hands. For this treatment technique you only require a coloured spotlight, or light box with a colour filter or even an ordinary coloured light bulb which you can obtain from a good lighting shop.

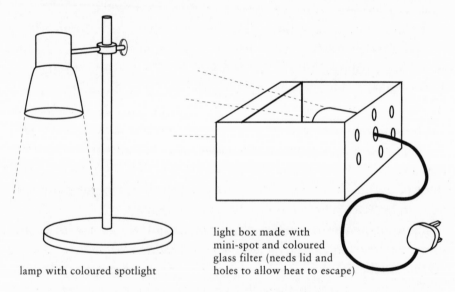

lamp with coloured spotlight

light box made with
mini-spot and coloured
glass filter (needs lid and
holes to allow heat to escape)

When you give colour light treatment with a colour lamp, make sure it is not too near the body as lamps give off a certain amount of heat. The light can also be focused on the appropriate area of the body while a massage or other treatment is given. Make sure you time the light treatment so it is not more than ten minutes as your client will feel uncomfortable if the lights are left on too long, and if this happens it will indicate that the aura is saturated with that particular colour energy.

Exact length of time for colour treatments depends on the severity of the problem. It is not the length of time that is important as the wave-length of colour vibration being sent. You only need to give the treatment long enough to send the colour vibration into the energetic system so it can act as a catalyst and start the healing process. In this respect colour therapy is like Homeopathy, whereby the potency and not the amount of the medicine is important. So it is the frequency or quality of the colour and not the amount that affects the healing.

Orange light can be used on the chest as it helps open the chest thus aiding breathing, but red can inflame and raise the heart beat too high, so do not use red above the solar-plexus. If you wish to treat the patient for emotional, mental or spiritual imbalances the safest way is to direct colour energy through the chakras. Red and orange are powerful colours and it is better to send these through the feet, rather than direct them on to top chakras. Colour can be focused on the soles of the feet at any stage of an aromatherapy treatment.

COLOUR REFLEXOLOGY USING OILS

Reflexology is an ancient therapy which is believed to have originated in China some 5000 years ago, when pressure therapies were commonly used to correct energy fields in the body. The ancient Egyptians, who also had a sophisticated system of colour therapy and aromatherapy used reflexology. All these healing methods were portrayed in colourful paintings on the walls of their tombs.

Reflexologists regard the foot as a mirror of the body, the left foot repre-senting the left side and the right foot the right side. Illness which is really energy imbalance, shows up as tender spots on the reflex areas which relate to the problem. Treatment of different conditions is by massage and pressure applied to the reflex areas on the feet, which clear the energy channels ending at these points. The organs and glands through which the energy channels run can be treated in this way, as can different emotional and mental problems.

In most complementary therapies, the body's energetic system is considered the basis of good health. Imbalances in the vital energy, or light energy, creates blocks which prevent this life giving force flowing freely through us. In order to be in good health at all levels a therapist needs to restore the flow of the white light, which contains all the colour vibrations, so that they can pass freely through the energetic field or aura.

The purpose of colour reflexology is to bring the patient back into harmony, through balancing the energy system throughout their being so that they become whole. The colour and aroma vibrations act as a catalysts which accelerate our own healing mechanisms so that we can become healthy and happy individuals. Through reflexology we can introduce the energy of colour and aroma into the etheric body to harmonise and balance the energetic system. Directing colour energy onto the chakras on the foot, the vibrations travel to the organs, glands and areas of the body with a sympathetic resonance. As healing vibrations penetrate to all parts of our being, we can not only treat physical ailments, but also mental and emotional problems. The vibrations of colour and aroma are the active ingredient of this therapy and reflexology the carrier or means of applying it.

A direct way of sending colour energy with the hands is by applying acupressure to the spinal reflex. You can also place a drop of essential oil on your thumb, and other fingers where appropriate. If you are not familiar with the chakra points on the foot, it is a good idea to massage essential oils and direct colours onto the solar-plexus reflex which is found in the centre of the sole of the foot. The solar-plexus, acts as the principal energy junction station directing energy to the chakras which require it. Lightly massage the solar-plexus area in the centre of the sole of the foot in circular movements with your thumbs or you can use a colour reflexology torch or crystal onto which a drop of essential oil has been placed.

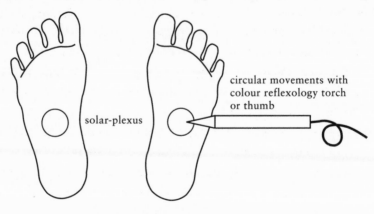

solar-plexus

circular movements with colour reflexology torch or thumb

When using reflexology combined with colour and aroma you should apply a steady light pressure to the reflex point. It is not your aim to make your patient tolerate more pain, for colour and aroma vibrations penetrate into their system once the point has been activated. It is the pattern of energy and not the strength of the pressure you apply which has the healing effect. Some colour reflexologists use a light instrument to activate the reflexes and to send colour energy through them to the corresponding areas. A drop of essential oil can be placed on the end of a colour reflexology torch which activates the foot reflex with light.

In colour reflexology one does not only treat the reflex points, but can send colour energy to larger areas of the foot which correspond to different areas of your life on an emotional, mental and spiritual level. It is also possible to send colour energy through the entire sole of the foot using light instruments in the same way as you do using the palms of your hands. For this treatment technique you require a coloured spotlight, or light box with a colour filter or even an angle poise light to which you have fitted a coloured light bulb.

When working with colour vibrations on the feet, a therapist often becomes sensitive to the colours and aromas in the aura of the person on whom they are working. Sometimes you will be able to tune in to the colours needed and channel these through your hands while working. You will also find that you develop the ability to treat the reflexes intuitively, feeling which ones are over-energised and which ones are under-energised.

SOLARISING BASE OILS

It is well known that due to their photo-sensitivity, essential oils should be kept away from sunlight. This is why essential oils are most commonly sold in dark brown bottles and stored in a dark, cool place. Colour aromatherapy recognises that the potency and healing qualities of the oils can be accelerated and enhanced by instilling the oil with colour energy of a sympathetic frequency. In order to do this without affecting the healing qualities, it is possible to energise the base (carrier) oil of a blend, rather than the essential oil itself.

By solarising carrier oils, which do not degrade when exposed to sunlight, it is possible to improve their potency and ability to absorb and disperse vibrational energy. Carrier oils should be placed in clear glass bottles on a window sill or out of doors in the direct sunlight for several hours and it does not matter if it is cloudy, as long as there is good natural light. There is no exact length of time for leaving the oils in the sun and you will need to use your intuition or a pendulum to dowse the correct length of time required.

Most base oils do, however, have a slight colour bias. Some are pale yellow, green or brown and it is a good idea to choose your base oil which suits the colour healing qualities you wish to instil. If you wish to mix a blend reflecting several different colours, try to choose a colourless or lightly coloured carrier oil, like some Sweet Almond or Grapeseed.

Green base oils, such as avocado or olive provide an overall healing medium, and are suitable for any type of colour blend. Sunflower oil, and peanut and safflower oil provide a good base for a yellow essential oil blend and for a mixture of violet and yellow ray oils. Carrot oil reflects the orange ray as does wheatgerm and sesame oil which contain both the orange and golden ray. Apricot and Peach Kernel oils reflect a more gentle and nurturing vibration reflected in their pale pinky-yellow colouring. These make good carrier oils for an essential oil blend which reflects the pink and green colour vibrations. The paler the oil, the more light energy it contains and the more it will harmonise with the higher colour vibrations and Yin essential oils.

Another method of solarising essential oils is by placing the prepared essential oil in a clear bottle which is placed under a coloured glass pyramid. When the oil is charged with the colour energy, it is poured into a normal brown dosage bottle. It is also possible to put the oil blend directly into a coloured glass bottle. Choose red for an energising blend, blue for a sedating one and green for a balancing mixture.

If the oil blend is to be used within a couple of weeks, for instance as a treatment for massage or as a bath oil, it can be kept in the coloured glass bottle. This is fine if it is put on a bathroom shelf or kept in a cabinet in a massage or therapy room in a cool place. It is important to make sure it is not exposed to direct sunlight.

The great energising qualities of pyramids have been recognised since ancient times. By placing a healing remedy or aromatic blend under a colour pyramid, its healing properties are increased and it becomes a powerful transmitter of light energy. If you wish to make a pyramid, you can use either coloured perspex or glass. I prefer glass as it is a natural product which has vibrations which are in tune with our own rhythms. The base of a glass pyramid should be nine inches square and the angle of the side 61 degrees. The height will be approximately 6 inches. This gives you the exact proportions used in the Great Pyramid of Giza.

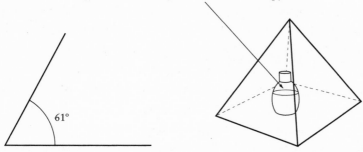

place oil in clear glass container under pyramid

61°

If you do not wish to buy glass pyramids made specifically for this purpose you can use colour filters which are available from reputable Colour Therapy schools.

Names of Colour Therapy schools are available from: International Association for Colour Therapy, P.O. Box 3, Potters Bar, Hertfordshire, EN6 3ET, U.K.

When mixing essential oils into a base oil put 1 drop of essential oil to 5 ml base oil, for facial blends. For body blends, add up to 3 drops to 5 ml base oil.

COLOUR AROMA MASSAGE

Colour-charged oil blends are perfect for massage and aromatherapy work. You can complement these treatments with the use of coloured lamps, the colour of the therapy room, the colour of the towels and your own clothing.

Using an infra-red lamp or coloured spotlight can also provide healing qualities which will reinforce your massage or treatment. If you have a movable light, you can also focus this on different areas of the body or chakras as you work. For instance if you are performing a lymphatic drainage on the legs, yellow light focused on the back of the legs will help move and cleanse the lymph nodes and glands.

You can massage a particular chakra in which case you mix up an appropriate oil blend for this chakra and its complementary pair. If you decide to stimulate and balance all the chakras, you will need to mix up a three oil blend to give a balance of colour energy for the bottom, middle and top chakras. (ie. it should contain a bottom, middle and top note reflecting the red, green and violet colour vibration).

COLOUR-AROMA LAMPS AND DIFFUSERS

Room diffusers are one of the most popular ways of enjoying the benefits of essential oils in the home and work place. By combining coloured light with the burning of oils, the energy in the room becomes more pervasive and the benefit to the occupants is increased. The synergy of healing energy will be directed through the eyes and nose as well as the etheric body of the people who move through the space.

A simple way of combining colour and aroma in a room diffuser is to use a light bulb ring made of unglazed ceramic. Place the diffuser on the light bulb when it is cold and switched off, then place a few drops of essential oils on the ring and place it over a light bulb. In Colour – Aromatherapy, you do exactly the same, but place the ring over a coloured light bulb. The glowing colour energy from the light bulb will combine with the oils and the heat will diffuse the vibrations throughout the room.

Another way of combining colour aroma in a room diffuser is by purchasing or commissioning a potter to make you a colour-aroma lamp. This lamp is partly a light and partly an oil burner. It needs to be quite large so that a standard bulb can be placed in the lamp holder. Above this the bowl containing water and your essential oils is placed. The heat from the lamp causes the water and oil mixture to gently evaporate. You do have to make sure the light bulb is near enough the bottom of the bowl for it to be heated sufficiently.

The lamp should be thrown in the round and can be a cylinder or gently curved and wide enough to get your hand inside. A bowl with a lip needs to be made to fit over the top of the opening. This needs to be removable so that you can change the light bulb. Alternatively, a large cut – out shape should be made in the side of the lamp which allows you access to the light bulb. Remember you need to see the colour of the light, but viewing the light bulb completely is not as attractive.

Cut out decorative shapes like stars, moons, circles, flowers etc from the sides so that the coloured light shines out. These lamps make wonderful bedside lights as well as decorative pieces in a sitting room, therapy room, work place or office. The beauty is that they are safe, having no open flame, and are excellent in places where there are children or animals present.

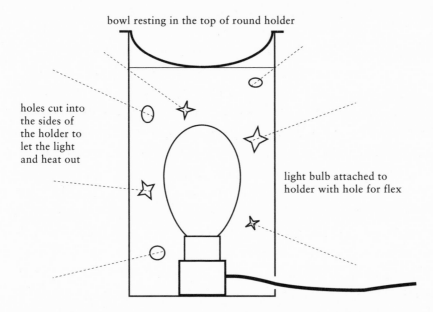

bowl resting in the top of round holder

holes cut into the sides of the holder to let the light and heat out

light bulb attached to holder with hole for flex

The following guide to the use of therapeutic lights is for colour-aroma lamp and for general irradiation light in the therapy room. (Coloured light bulbs or spotlight). Also included are tips for using a colour crystal torch, or directional coloured spotlight.

Healing with light from the visible spectrum is entirely safe as long as you make sure that strong light is not directed into the eyes or a powerful lamp is not in close contact with the body. It is only light from the invisible part of the spectrum, for instance infra-red and ultra-violet light, that is able to burn living tissue. We should not, however, underestimate the powerful and penetrating effect of light therapy and if you find someone is uncomfortable, stop the light treatment. This may happen when a person is sensitive to a certain colour or the chakra is saturated with the colour energy. Switch the colour treatment to the complementary colour, which will help balance the energy vibration. Complementary colour energies have the capacity of seeking a balanced energy level, ensuring there is not too much or too little of either vibration in the system.

THERAPEUTIC QUALITIES OF LIGHT

Pink Light
This is particularly useful in a therapy room or bedroom, as pink light has muscle relaxant qualities by increasing the supply of blood to the muscles. Pink contains the stimulating and releasing action of the red ray, although pink has a much gentler action. This warming and loving colour should be used to encourage love and nurturing. Pink light is especially useful when one is feeling lonely, unloved, rejected or grieving. Shone on the heart chakra, it provides healing of the emotions and connects one with universal and unconditional love vibrations. It is a good colour for children too.

Orange Light
Orange is a warming and stimulating colour. It creates an atmosphere of happiness and vitality. Orange energy boosts the immune system and is an excellent tonic. It also has a releasing action, helping move body fluids around the body. Use orange light to combat depression by allowing deep-seated emotions to surface.

Yellow Light
Yellow warms and energises without creating heat in the body. It has an affinity with the stomach and spleen and has a cleansing and purgative action. This vibration helps remove toxins from the blood stream and lympthatics and can be of assistance in an aromatherapy treament when directed onto these glands. When focused on the solar-plexus chakra or foot reflex, yellow helps remove energy blocks in the emotional and mental bodies. Use it to build up self-confidence and self-worth, and to dispel fears of the mind.

Red Light

Red light is usually associated with stimulation and particularly sexual passion. Red light is indeed very warming and stimulates the release of adrenalin, sexual appetite and muscular activity. Red light strengthens the blood supply to the heart by raising the pulse and the heart beat. Only focus red light on the lower part of the body, as red energy is very powerful and has some contra-indications. (Do not use on anyone with high blood pressure or a heart condition). Red light shone on the feet can stimulate life-force energy through the body, and can be used if someone has collapsed, fainted or lost consciousness. Make sure you also call for medical assistance.

Green Light

Green light is very cooling and soothing but is not good when you wish to read or concentrate on a task. The benefits of green light are greatest when you have your eyes closed and is excellent for the treatment of stress. Use green light to relax and unwind, especially after a hot bath or when you practise some meditation or relaxation technique. Green candles to which a couple of drops of essential oil has been added is good for calming and balancing one's emotions. Green light speeds up the body's own healing mechanism so is good for recuperation. It has also been found that green light speeds up the healing of fractured bones, sprains and strains.

Blue Light

Blue light is exceptionally soothing and cooling. Use it in hot rooms, or when you are suffering from anger or a fever or any ailment where you have a high temperature. Blue light helps one sleep and calms the mind but the eyes find it difficult to focus in blue light so it is not good for reading or when you are doing an exacting task. A blue light next to the bed can help calm hyperactive children and it is also good for soothing childhood diseases like chickenpox, measles, etc. It is especially useful in cases of sunstroke and burns, bringing relief from pain and speeding up the healing process. Blue has a constrictive action (stemming the flow of blood and so useful for treating cuts, bruises and nose bleeds.)

Violet Light

The balancing effect Violet light has on the psyche has resulted in it being used successfully in many mental institutions to help people with obsessive behaviour patterns and neuroses. At home a purple light bulb can help harmonise one's mental and emotional state. It can also aid meditation and balance the left and right hand side of the brain connecting you to your creativity and spirituality. Violet light should only be used for short periods of time for specific balancing treatments. Use violet light directly on the body to purify the blood. It is especially useful when focused on varicose veins.

AROMA COLOUR BATHS

One of the best ways to make use of this powerful but subtle combination of colour and aroma is at home in the bath. The idea is not a new one, and the ancient system of Solar-ray healing in India still recommends therapeutic colour baths to-day. In India where it is warm with plenty of natural sunlight, baths are placed on the flat roof of the clinic and covered with sheets of coloured glass or coloured silk cloth. Lying in one of these baths in the sunlight, provides a wonderful colour treatment which leaves one feeling energised and full of vitality.

We should remember that a hot bath not only cleanses the skin, it also cleanses the aura from negative vibrations which you may have picked up during the day, from other people and the polluted environment. We can make use of this receptive time by making sure the aura is recharged by absorbing positive vibrations of colour and aroma which will energise and re-balance the energetic system. As a hot bath can deplete the aura leaving you vulnerable to outside vibrations, an evening bath allows time for your aura to re-charge.

The simplest way of having an aroma colour bath is by using an essential oil blend in the bath water, while simultaneously taking in coloured light vibrations through the eyes. Candles are particularly good for providing soft and nourishing light while bathing. The colour of the glowing candle provides natural colour vibrations which will enhance the action of the bath oils. Other ways of providing coloured light while bathing are by putting a coloured light bulb into the bathroom light. Pink or peachy toned lights in a bathroom work best, as these make the skin glow and provide loving and emotionally supporting colour vibrations. Fluorescent or striplights should be avoided at all times as these emit pulsing flickers of light vibrations which can make one ill. A bathroom blind can also filter coloured light into the room during daylight. Blue or green is cooling and relaxing and is restful to the mind. Pink or peach is soothing on the emotions and relaxing to the physical body.

A colour aroma bath can be made by literally colouring the bath water into which corresponding essential oils are added. Natural plant colouring which does not affect the skin can also make a gentle colour bath. Beetroot juice which has been well diluted, so that it doesn't stain,) produces a lovely pink bath, while chamomile flower water is a soft pale yellow. Boiled peppermint leaves colours a bath a pale green.

Perhaps the most wonderful way of having a colour aroma bath is by using fresh flowers in the bath water. A handful of rose petals, violets, chamomile flowers, herbs or lavender can create a delicately perfumed bath with colour energy. You could add a few drops of floral water or essential oils of the appropriate flowers as well. You do, however, need to visually see the colour of the flowers in the bath, so tying them in a muslin bag is not a good idea if you wish to reap the benefits of colour as well as the benefits of the aroma.

If fresh flowers are not available blue, green, orange or pink cake colouring can also be used but it is not recommended to have a red bath, as most people associate this colour with blood! You can purchase colour baths made from natural plant materials from a Colour Therapy supplier as well as some natural cosmetic companies.

COLOUR COMPRESSES

Herbal compresses and those using essential oils have been found to be extremely effective in relieving a host of physical ailments. You will need to get a selection of coloured flannels, warm colours for drawing poultices on boils and tension and strains, and cool colours for inflammation, headaches and swellings.

Fill a basin with hot water and saturate a coloured flannel in the water. Now pour a few drops of essential oils into the water and squeeze out the flannel and place over the area to be treated. When the flannel cools down to blood temperature, repeat. You can also make cold compresses in the same way or alternate hot and cold on strained ligaments and tendons.

You can make coloured dressing in a similar way, but with the addition of a coloured bandage. Burns have been treated very successfully with blue bandages and lavender oil. Blue is a pain healer, cooling and encourages the growth of scar tissue. Green helps fractures knit, and promotes normal cell growth. Yellow is good for purifying and for many skin conditions.

Another way of making a colour compress is by using healing flowers or leaves of a therapeutic colour (check the flowers or leaves are not poisonous), directly on the wound or area requiring healing. You can also wrap healing colours around the bottle of essential oil blend which you are going to use as the compress. I have wrapped Violet leaves around an essential oil mixture of Chamomile and Juniper and found it a wonderful healing blend for soothing aching and swollen joints.

Tansy, which vibrates on the yellow ray, makes a good poultice which can be applied externally on varicose veins, swellings, bruises, styes and eye inflammations. Blue cornflowers make a soothing eyebath for chronic and acute eye inflammations as well as corneal ulcers. Foxglove leaves can be used as a remedy to ease pain, swellings and tumours. Warmed in hot water and placed on the forehead, they relieve headaches and a leaf warmed and rolled is soothing for earache.

COLOURED SPRAY MISTS

Spray mists are an old fashioned way of using floral waters or aromatic water either as a perfume or a spray which can be used as an air freshener or linen mist. Spray mists are very economical to make and have many beneficial uses for healing of the body, mind and spirit.

To make an oil spray mist you will need:

- A clear plastic or glass bottle with a pump action spray. You should be able to buy one at a good chemist or pharmacy. Alternatively you can use a coloured glass perfume bottle with a pump spray. You can use a plant spray for larger quantities which are useful to keep in the bathroom.
- Essential oils

- Warm purified or distilled water. Spring or mineral water is not suitable as these have live bacteria present which may in time cause the spray mist to go off.
- Vegetable or natural colouring. Aromatherapy suppliers can supply you with natural food colouring.

Simply put the water into the bottle and add a few drops of harmonising essential oils and shake thoroughly. Use 4 drops of essential oil to a half pint of water (250ml). Add a few drops of colouring until the desired colour is reached. Remember the colour will act in unity with the oils, so the colour must be in sympathetic resonance.

You can use the spray mist as a body perfume after a bath or shower, or to refresh you when you are tired. Keep a spray at work for a quick freshen and pick-me-up. In the home you can keep the spray in the bathroom as a room freshener. It is best to use anti-bacterial oils with a blue or violet colouring, and this type of spray is excellent in a room if you have a cold, cough or flu. As a linen spray, a rose pink colour with a mixture of Palmarosa or a pale lavender hue with Lavender oil gives a delicate and long lasting aroma to sheets and towels. Do not spray a colour spray directly onto the linen, just spray a little into the linen cupboard.

On an emotional and spiritual level, a colour spray mist cleanses negative vibrations from a room especially where there has been smoking, drinking or an argument. A therapy room is the perfect place to use a spray mist. Use it to cleanse the therapy or massage couch of vibrations so that they do not transfer from one person to another.

COLOUR-AROMA BREATHING

Breathing is essential to life, for it is from the air that we extract oxygen to feed our physical body and brain and prana to feed our energetic system. Although our breathing is automatic, many people do not reap the benefits from deep, slow breathing. Many problems related to low energy levels could be easily solved if we learned to breathe properly, and many imbalances occurring deep within our system could be redressed with conscious use of breathing techniques.

The air is full of forces of light, colour, sound, aroma and electro-magnetic energy. We breathe in these vibrations every minute of our lives so the quality of the air will affect our quality of life and our energy levels. The breath itself is coloured, and we continuously breathe into ourselves the colour vibrations of the people, places and objects around us.

Each of our chakras accumulates negativity by our thoughts and actions so that if someone is depressed, or has been smoking, they will breathe out grey or brown energy and their dirt will become super-imposed on our energy centres. We should aim to breathe in the colours we need and breath out the dark, dirty colours which are polluting us on the inside. By learning to breathe properly we can learn to heal ourselves, the deep breath penetrating deep into our body and mind. Those who have practised certain types of yoga, metaphysics or spiritual healing techniques have used colour breathing with excellent results.

By learning how to colour breathe, you can direct colour, together with a source of life energy contained in the breath, to any part of your body, your glands, organs, even your face and eyes, or you can direct it to protect inanimate objects like your home and belongings. By also applying aromatherapy to these areas by massage, baths, compresses or diffusion you are able to replace negative vibrations with positive ones which are in keeping with your own internal colours and harmonies.

It is not only proper nutrition and physical exercise but proper thinking that promotes good health. Many complementary medical practices recognise the power of mind waves, in contributing to the healing process and in many clinics serious illnesses like cancer, M.E. and AIDS, involve both aromatherapy and colour visualisations in their treatment programme. Our thoughts are vibrations which spread out around us in space, much like the ripples in a pond and so our thought waves can be used for positive vibrational healing reinforce the effects of colour and aroma. Many methods of psychotherapy can help us identify and release deep-seated internal emotional blocks which affect our health, but colour breathing and visualisation helps us unblock these channels psychically.

A simple way to inhale colour and aroma is to place a drop of essential oil on a carefully chosen coloured handkerchief or cloth and inhale the scent. The effects are uncomplicated, immediate and can be done anywhere and at any time. When travelling, I always keep a Lavender handkerchief onto which I have placed a couple of drops of lavender, Juniper or Tea-tree oil in my pocket. Before a lecture or an interview, I inhale a yellow-ray oil like basil or Niaouli, Lime or Grapefruit to relax nervous tension and clear my head.

Aroma can also be inhaled by steam into which clearing essential oils like Eucalyptus and Pine have been placed and if you were to focus your mind on deep blue, the potency of the treatment would be that much greater.

Using colour visualisation is not merely a technique with instant visible results; it has to be understood and practised regularly. We need to focus our minds on a particular colour and positive blueprint will be picked up through our etheric body. If we consistently programme our blueprint on a daily basis, the message will get through with very tangible results. Like learning to drive or ride a bicycle, we need to practice consistently before we internalise the process and do it automatically.

Linda Clark and Yvonne Martine in their wonderful book *Health, Youth and Beauty through Colour Breathing* tell us that, if we want a happy life, we must think happy thoughts. If we want a prosperous life, we must think prosperous thoughts. If we want a loving life, we must think loving thoughts. Whatever we send out mentally or verbally will come back to us in like form. We must, however, think these thoughts sincerely and not for our own gain, as you cannot deceive yourself, or deceit will be mirrored back to you.

Here are some essential guidelines that are needed for colour breathing to work well:

1. Practise colour breathing and positive visualisations in a light airy room, preferably in the early morning or sunset. This is the time when the most prana or Ch'i energy fills the air. Place some harmonious oils in a room diffuser and let the aroma pervade the space where you will be practising colour breathing.
2. Visualise only what you wish to happen for your own highest good. Negative thoughts imprint themselves too. So if you are constantly expecting the worst, you are blocking out good vibrations from your system.
3. Work out a Colour-related positive affirmation and repeat it consistently as well as daily. This is equivalent to a new programme of software for the mind, changing negative thought patterns into positive ones. So if you are prone to say things like ... It always happens to me, or I am no good, ugly, stupid, unlucky etc. these thoughts will be constantly reinforced in your system.

4. Thought is vibration and a stronger vibration will work better than a weak one, so concentrate and visualise strongly. The mind needs to be focused in order to send out pure and resonant thought waves. These strong vibrations will over-ride the mass of worried and confused thoughts swirling around our heads.
5. Add colour to your visualisations and affirmations to reinforce the vibrational effects. Use colour affirmations to focus on qualities you want to enhance.

MEDITATION

No matter what your philosophy of life, meditation can provide us with a means for developing alertness of mind, a greater ability to concentrate, reduced stress levels and help us find more enjoyment and purpose in life.

The combination of high vibrational frequencies of light and aroma during meditation, enables us to still our busy conscious mind, providing a focus for our thoughts and open a channel enabling us to connect to the divine within us. By freeing ourselves of unwanted compulsions, addictions and stress we are able to take back our power and focus ourselves towards more beneficial and productive things. The result is a feeling of well-being and peace, something we all need in the world to-day.

Colour and aroma also heighten our awareness linking us to the spiritual forces within and around us. As colour and aroma exists on both a physical and subtle plane, they are the perfect tools to provide us with a link to other dimensions. Different perfumes work upon our spiritual bodies in different ways. The transformative effects of the aroma of Frankincense and Lavender work through the violet flame of purification, raising our internal vibrations so that we can connect to higher realms. Meditating with certain colours and aromas can help connect us with our guardian angel and inner guides giving us a glimpse of the radiance of the great light beings who exist in higher planes of existence.

The simplest way of using colour and aroma for meditation is by contemplating a beautiful flower, inhaling the perfume of the flower before placing it on a table in front of you. The beautiful symmetry of shape and colour will draw the mind into the mystic centre helping to unify and raise the consciousness to higher levels. Often people burn incense or joss sticks in the room while they are meditating. This is an ancient practise and is very important for cleansing the space in which you are sitting from negative and harmful vibrations. If you decide to burn joss sticks, it is a good idea to make sure you buy a product made from the best quality ingredients. A good quality incense stick is hand rolled using essential oils, beeswax and flower pollen.

The best form of colour to introduce for meditation is the living natural light of a candle. There are hundreds of beautifully coloured candles to choose from and many of them are scented with essential oils. Choose the shape and colour of the candle to soothe, balance or inspire you, using your intuition or a pendulum to dowse the colour and aroma you need.

Colour breathing can be very successfully used to aid contemplation and meditation techniques for thousands of years by followers of many different religious and spiritual practises all over the world. Deep breathing is the key to meditation as it helps us to relax the body and mind and extract life-force energy, also known as Prana or Ch'i, from the air. Green colour breathing is best for slowing us down so we become sensitive to vibrations coming from within. Green energy works through the parasympathetic nervous system inducing the lungs to relax, thus drawing in more air. The more slowly and deeply we breathe the more relaxed we feel.

Deep midnight blue (Indigo) helps us open the third eye, and develops our inner vision so we can come to know and understand ourselves. At the end of a meditation session, breathing in red energy, linked to the 'Kundalini' fire at the base of the spine, charges our aura with energy leaving us full of vitality.

Aroma	Colour	Aid to meditation
Hyacinth	blue	useful for self-hypnosis techniques linking to the right side of the brain and feminine side
Hyssop	violet	purifies the air and sacred places
Angelica	silver/gold	fortifies the female spirit, provides flexibility and gentleness. Opens channel of light which connects to the angelic realms.

Aroma	Colour	Aid to meditation
Silver Fir Needle	silver	provides focus for the third eye and the pineal gland
Vetivert	gold	oil of tranquillity has a calming action on the mind. Opens our connection with your internal sun, your 'soul'.
Violet	purple	pain-killing properties, anaesthetising and narcotic action on the mind, slowing down brain waves and promoting a feeling of brotherhood of mankind.
Sandalwood	blue	frees the soul bringing peace, acceptance and understanding.
Patchouli	peach	sedating through the ground connection, channels creative and healing energy downwards, frees the mind of restrictive patterns and attitudes preventing spiritual progress.
Jasmine	deep pink	releases fear and guilt, especially from past lives. Purity of spirit allows for connection to angelic forces.
Rose	red	dissolves grief and pain from the heart allowing universal love to flow and growth to take place.
Lavender	purple	stabilises physical, etheric and astral body, soothes the spirit. Calms and purifies, transformative and raises consciousness.

FRESH FLOWERS

Nature has provided us with a perfect union of colour and aroma in plants themselves. A bowl of cut flowers can provide both a beautiful array of colours and perfumes which permeates the room and our aura with healing vibrations. We should not forget the more subtle effects of herbs and leaves, and a jug filled with fresh green herbs on a table can awaken our senses and leave us feeling cleansed and refreshed. Receiving a bunch of flowers is still named as the most desirable gift by men and women alike, and so understanding the potential for healing energy carried in a bunch of flowers, we can give to others a doubly wonderful gift.

One of the main reasons we send flowers is when someone is ill. Light healing pastels of pink, blue and violet fragrances are better for people who are extremely ill. These flowers usually have delicate aromas, which are soothing and healing. When the person is feeling stronger an uplifting bunch of orange and gold flowers will feed them nourishing energy needed for full recuperation.

For those special events, like Birthdays or passing exams, an array of strongly scented and brightly coloured flowers can reinforce an air of celebration and bring with them a radiant glow of joy and happiness.

Roses have always been associated with love, but we should think more carefully about the type of love vibrations we wish to give with flowers. Red roses, with their deep lush scent, are linked to physical love and desire. Orange and yellow roses send messages of upliftment and rejoicing in love. Often their fresh apple or fruity scents bring renewed awakening where love has faded or been subject to obstructions. Deep pink roses give off an unconditional love vibration which lets the receiver know that you love them without expecting anything in return. Salmon pink is also the colour of divine love relating to all humanity rather than individuals. The paler the colour of the rose, the more pure the love, so white roses reveal a love which is pure and spiritual.

Scent	Rose	Colour
Apple	'Francois Juranville'	pink
	'Paul Transon'	copper-orange
	'Rene Andre'	apricot – orange
	'Silver Moon'	
Cloves	'Blush Noisette'	lilac-pink
Musk	'Pauls's Himalayan Musk'	blush – pink
	'Day Break'	yellow opening to light yellow
	'Penelope'	creamy-white
Lemony	'Mme Hardy'	white, blush tinted in bud

Scent	Rose	Colour
Myrrh	'Constance Spry'	clear rose pink
	'Cressida'	apricot pink
Orange	'The Garland'	creamy – salmon
	'Veilchenblau'	dark magenta
Primrose	'Adelaide d'Orleans'	creamy – white
	'Debutante'	clear rose pink
Sweet Pea	'Mme Gregoire Staechelin'	coral pink with crimson overtones
	'Vanity'	deep pink
Raspberry	'Cerise Bouquet'	cerise pink

Read up on the secret language of flowers, and when choosing flowers, make sure the colour and scent carry your special vibrational message.

SLEEPY-TIME PILLOWS

Herbal pillows have ancient origins but were made popular by the Victorians. They were lovingly made and filled with dried soothing and relaxing herbs. Essential oils are perfect for infusing into herbal pillows, especially when the pillow also contains sleep inducing colour energy. We can use sleepy-time pillows not only for their sleep inducing qualities, but as a tool for allowing colour and aroma to permeate our aura while we are most sensitive to these healing vibrations.

Choose a natural fabric coloured blue or green to relax the mind and breathing. It could be decorated with a floral pattern or with shapes and forms taken from nature. You could also include a soft peach or pink in the design which would help soothe the emotions. Fill the pillow with a mixture of hops, lavender, valerian, lemon verbena or other pacifying herbs, adding a few drops of essential oils which have a sympathy with the green, blue or pink ray.

Place under your regular pillow or inside the pillowcase making sure it is white or off-white in colour allowing the natural colour energy of the sleepy pillow to filter through. As both colour vibrations and aroma can be absorbed into our system at night, when our sensitivity to these subtle energies are at their highest, we can use colour and aroma vibrations to help us link to our unconscious mind. Sleepy-time pillows have been found to be extremely useful for anyone wishing to recall their dreams. Often our dreams release energy blocks which we suppress during our waking hours and if we pay attention to our dreams they can be a wonderful aid for personal development and inner growth. The following essential oils and colours can assist us while we are asleep in the following ways.

Oil	Colour	Healing through dreams
Bay Laurel	Blue	Prophetic dreams
Clary Sage	Magenta/Orchid	Vivid Dreams and their recall
Melissa	Pink/Green	Past Life recall through dreaming
Sandalwood	Blue	Helps release anxieties which cause recurring dreams
Yarrow	Deep blue	Self-development through dreams by seeing our life clearly and from a different perspective
Neroli	Peach/Cream	Inner communication and past life healing during a deep sleep. Wake refreshed.

HEALING WITH CRYSTALS AND GEMSTONES

Everything in the universe is made up of the same basic elements which form the basis of our planetary system and all living things. Plants have a strong connection to the earth, and as a result have an affinity with certain rocks and gemstones. We, too, need minerals for life and health and are grounded to the earth through gravitational forces. The planets exert a strong energy on the earth, which affects the growth and development of plants, and the moon particularly can stimulate or retard the growth of plants through its strong pull on the tides and water on the earth. It is, therefore, not so strange that we can make use of the energy forces which flow through gemstones and plants as part of a healing treatment.

The healing power of gemstones and crystals has been known since ancient times. Crystals are alive, pulsating with energy and are able to absorb, hold and reflect colour energy. The pyramid structure of the crystal together with its ability to absorb and amplify white light makes them the most highly evolved of all minerals. Clear quartz crystals have the capacity to absorb, hold and amplify electro-magnetic energy and for this reason they were used during the Second World War in crystal radio sets.

Crystals have the capacity to change the vibratory rate within our physical and subtle bodies, so dispersing energy blocks and restoring a balance and flow of energy through the chakras. The white light entering the crystal energises it and the prismatic internal formation of the crystal amplifies the rays which are then released through its pyramid shaped point. This is why it is most important you align the crystal in the direction you wish the energy to flow.

By using clear quartz crystals, we can direct healing vibratory patterns of the plant to different parts of our energetic system. As you are working with the subtle bodies, you first have to select an essential oil or make a blend or oils which will create a positive energy pattern which will be absorbed into the chakras. You may decide to use an oil for its energising, releasing, balancing or healing qualities or you can create a blend of oils which will work on various levels simultaneously.

There are many ways you can combine essential oils and crystal healing. Firstly you can lay the crystals in a pattern around the body, while you give a massage treatment. This will assist with cleansing, balancing and energising the chakras and re-charging the auric field. Secondly you can place a drop of essential oil on the point of the crystal and use the crystal to move energy in the etheric body, by moving it in circular or sweeping movements just above the physical body.

COLOUR AND GEMSTONE HEALING

Crystals reflect the transformative energy of white light which pervades our spiritual bodies, but often we need to unlock energy in the more dense vibrations of the physical, emotional and mental bodies. For moving energy on the physical plane, the healing vibrations of gemstones can prove very effective. Gemstones are less evolved than crystals and each stone is tuned in to a particular ray and has a particular function and purpose to serve.

Stones show changes in growth as layer upon layer of thousands of years give us the message that life is about change and evolution. The more transparent and reflective the stone, the purer the light frequency passing through it and the stronger the healing power. First anoint each chakra with a healing oil and then lay a gemstone of the corresponding colour directly on the energy centre. This will have the effect of energising and tuning the chakra to the healing colour frequency. You can also anoint the temples, hands and feet before laying on gemstones.

You can combine the healing power of gemstones with an aromatherapy treatment by first giving the massage and then laying the gemstones on the chakras for balancing at the end of the session for ten minutes or so. Often the stones will roll off the chakra, and if this happens do not replace them, for it indicates that the chakra is energised and the stone has completed its healing work.

For calming and balancing the physical body, choose green stones essential oils such as melissa or geranium. To balance the mental body use indigo and green stones with oils which are calming to the mind. In order to pacify the spiritual body use light blue stones such as blue topaz and sapphire and oils like Yarrow, Rosemary or Roman Chamomile.

If you wish to give a revitalising healing session, select orange stones for the physical, emerald green or royal blue for the mental and golden and rose-pink gems for the spiritual. Combine with essential oils which reflect these colours.

For an inspirational and stimulating gemstone treatment choose red and pink stones for the physical, yellow, gold and violet stones to stimulate the higher mind and violet stones to act on the spiritual bodies.

Many less evolved gemstones do not have stong healing vibrations, but can be used as 'touch stones' for it is by handling them that they impart their vibrations. Many good touchstones are green in colour as they give out a slow even pulse of energy. Place these stones near you in the home or office and pick them up when you feel the need. I like to place a drop of Geranium or Palmarosa oil on the touchstone to increase its healing qualities.

Colour energy	Gemstones	Healing qualities
White Light	Diamond	balances the whole aura
	Clear Rock Crystal	decrystalises energy blocks
	Opal	energises all chakras
Silver	Moonstone	promotes inner growth (feminine energy)
Black	Smoky Quartz	shield of protection
	Black tourmaline	Base chakra energiser
	Obsidian	Native American protective stone
Red	Ruby	actives the energy in the physical body, lifts passion to compassion
	Garnet	generative stimulant and circulation
Pink	Rose Quartz	love, feminine energy
	Pink Tourmaline (Rubellite)	balances heart so we accept love without judgement or expectations
	Watermelon Tourmaline	balances polarity in the body, and heart chakra (synergy of pink and green energy)
Orange	Carnelian	grounding, sacral chakra
	Coral	firmness and co-operation
	Pearl	transmutation through pain
	Amber	immune stimulant, releasing the past
Gold	Gold	wisdom
Yellow	Topaz	inspiration for the higher mind
	Citrine	dispels fears, and boosts endocrine system
	Amber (Yellow)	nourishes nervous system and brain

Colour energy	Gemstones	Healing qualities
Green	Emerald	revitalises the body
	Jade	overall healing and balancing, longevity
	Aventurine	calming touchstone
	Moss Agate	balancing touchstone
	Green Jasper	serenity touchstone
	Malachite	balances whole system
	Chrysoprase	sedative/tranquilliser
	Green Tourmaline	rejuvenates and regenerates
	Peridot	balances emotions
Turquoise	Turquoise	honouring physical body and protection
	Chrysocolla	helps us connect with nature
	Aquarmarine	clarity of vision
Blue	Sapphire	purification and pain healer
	Lapis Lazuli	instils high ideals and meditation
	Sodalite	purifying and curative
Indigo	Blue Topaz	creative energy
	Azurite	great healer and brings inner sight
	Fluorite	calms the nerves and brings wisdom
Violet	Amethyst	balances sexual polarity, dispels fears and anxieties
	Sugilite	divine love and self-acceptance

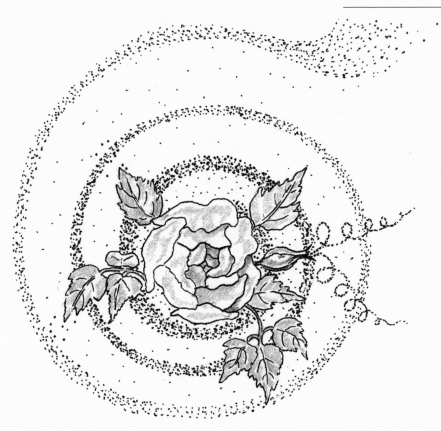

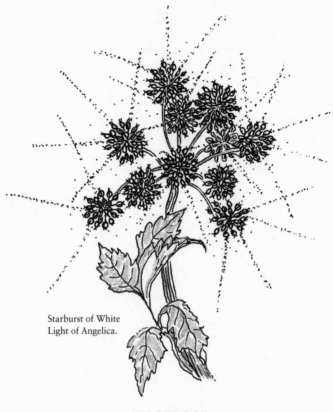

Starburst of White
Light of Angelica.

ANGELICA

ANGELICA ARCHANGELICA
Healing colours/s: white and pale yellow
Colour aroma treatment/s: colour massage, colour aroma bath, colour
breathing, colour spray mist, colour aroma lamp
Chakra affinity: heart
Life qualities: peace, spiritually opening, purity, harmony, fertility

Colour signature: Angelica, which is also known as 'angel's grass' is a
water-loving herb with strongly scented white flowers. The oil can be
made from either the roots and rhizomes or the fruit and seed and is
colourless to pale yellow but turns a deep yellow as it ages. Oil made
from the seeds carries yellow and green energy while that made from the
flowers is creamy-white. The yellow energy and acts as a tonic but with a
strong healing action while the white light lifts the soul and raises our consciousness levels. The ability of Angelica to connect us with our spiritual
nature confirms its ancient connections with the spirit world. The roots

have an affinity with water which gives Angelica its balancing and harmonising effect on the emotions. Its tall stately appearance and yellow energy gives it a strengthening quality, as it invigorates the lymphatic system and expelling poisons from the body. Yellow also works on the digestive system while the green energy harmonises with the respiratory system. The green ray in Angelica makes it link to the female aspect, encouraging the production of oestrogen and regulating menstruation.

Therapeutic uses	Aromatherapy	Colour therapy
Physical	cleanses the body, through lymphatic drainage and sweating	yellow through the feet
	eliminates toxins through the skin	yellow over abdomen
	good for indigestion, flatulence, dyspepsia, stomach ulcers, colic	yellow over stomach
	good for feverish colds, chronic bronchitis and pleurisy	yellow over chest
	female complaints, and fertility in both sexes	yellow over lower abdomen
Emotional	balances the emotions and good for moodiness	gold over the heart
Mental	good for mental stress and nervous exhaustion	gold over the head
Spiritual	strengthens the aura through emotional balance	white colour breathing
	peace through purity and love	white crystal healing and meditation

Precautions: Avoid during pregnancy, do not use on diabetics, some photo-toxicity.

Affirmations: With the white light in Angelica I create a channel for spiritual guidance.

ANISEED

PIMPINELLA ANISUM
Healing colours/s: orange and gold
Colour aroma treatment/s: Spray mists, colour compresses, colour aromatic cooking, colour aroma lamps, room diffusers, perfumes, colour breathing
Chakra affinity: sacral, hara
Life qualities: contentment, action-oriented, enthusiastic

Colour signature: The warm brown colouring of the seeds of this widely used spice gives Aniseed its colour signature. The delicate herb on which they grow has small feathery leaves and white flowers. The essential oil is spicy and sweet-scented, reminding one of warm, soporific late summer days. Its deep tap root gives Aniseed a strong earth connection and the orange ray reflected by this oil acts as a general tonic and is warming and freeing to the emotions. Its invigorating action is good for a tired mind, and the golden energy promotes clarity of thought, aids memory and is a good concentration aid. The colour orange activates the hara centre, the seat of power and self-confidence, and as Aniseed reflects this energy it has a releasing and opening effect making it good for the treatment of sexual problems and promoting sharing and caring relationships.

Therapeutic uses	Aromatherapy	Colour therapy
Physical	warming and a general tonic to the body	orange light to whole body
	use for nausea caused from nervousness	orange light to solar-plexus
	stimulates cardiac fatigue	orange to chest
	relieves breathing difficulties	orange to chest
	impotence and frigidity	orange to pelvic area

Emotional	warming and freeing action on the emotions	orange to sacral centre
	encourages tactile enjoyment and touch	orange to sacral centre
	promotes action and builds self-esteem	orange to sacral centre
Mental	invigorating to a tired mind	gold to solar-plexus
	brings sharpness to the mind	gold to solar-plexus
Spiritual	releases blocks in the astral body	gold to heart chakra
	helps us bring spirit into matter	gold to crown chakra

Precautions: Avoid during pregnancy. Can cause dermatitis, and in large doses is a narcotic.

Affirmations: With the orange ray in Aniseed I am free to enjoy the sensory pleasures of life.

BASIL

OCIMUM BASILICUM

Healing colours/s: yellow and violet
Colour aroma treatment/s: aroma spray mist, colour aroma lamp, colour breathing, colour compresses and poultices, solar charged water
Chakra affinity: solar-plexus and crown
Life qualities: optimism, cheerfulness, integrity, wholeness, balance

Colour signature: Basil is a lovely herb which is particularly favoured in France for its spicy and clear sweet fragrance. The plant is tender and has green soft oval leaves with purple-white flowers. The yellow and violet rays are equally present in Basil and work together on the endocrine system, mind and central nervous system giving the oils its cooling, uplifting and restorative qualities. The Chinese have used Basil since ancient times as a cure for epilepsy, and this makes sense when considering its colour signatures. The yellow and violet ray opens the crown chakra to allow vital energy into the system, while yellow strengthens the nerves through which the energy travels to other parts of the body. From the viewpoint of a holistic practitioner, epilepsy is caused by the blocking of vital energy, resulting in a seizure or fit. By removing the energy block and restoring the flow of energy through the chakras, which are linked to the nerves, vital energy can circulate freely once more.

Therapeutic uses	Aromatherapy	Colour therapy
Physical	congestive problems in the lungs, and respiratory tract, sinusitis, asthma, bronchitis, emphysema, influenza, whooping cough	yellow over lungs
	digestive disorders: vomiting, gastric spasm, nausea, hiccups, dyspepsia,	yellow over abdomen
	tonic and refreshing to the skin, insect bites,	yellow to the soles of the feet
	cleanses kidneys and intestines	yellow to lower abdomen
Emotional	for people of a nervous disposition, feeling vulnerable and afraid, hysteria	yellow to solar-plexus chakra
	helps assertiveness in shy people	yellow to solar-plexus chakra
Mental	stimulates mind, focusing, helps alertness, but over use results in sedation	yellow followed by violet to crown
Spiritual	promotes feelings of self-worth	yellow to solar-plexus chakra

Precautions: Avoid during pregnancy, can irritate the skin.

Affirmations: With the yellow ray in Basil, I am alert and ready for anything. The violet ray allows life force energy to flood my system, so every part of me is energised.

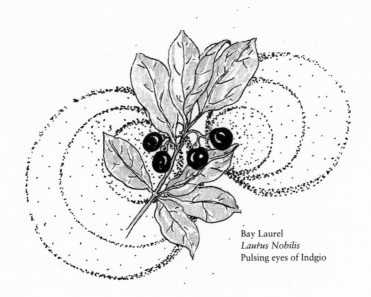

Bay Laurel
Laurus Nobilis
Pulsing eyes of Indgio

BAY LAUREL

LAURUS NOBILIS

Healing colours/s: indigo and green
Colour aroma treatment/s: perfumes, toiletries, colour room diffuser, solarised water, colour aroma bath, colour spray mist, colour compress
Chakra affinity: base, heart, throat, brow
Life qualities: wisdom, peace, protection, intuition, expression

Colour signature: The Bay tree is an ornamental evergreen, the leaves of which are often used in cooking and which has creamy-yellow flowers followed by blue-black berries. The essential oil is made from the dry leaf and branches and sometimes from the berries. Bay Laurel has a mixture of colour signatures, the main two being indigo and green linking to its two important qualities the first being a tonic and invigorating and the second being sedating. The red energy within indigo acts as an appetite stimulant and strengthens the digestion and reproductive system. The blue/black

111

berries give the bay its deep blue frequency which is linked to the throat and also the flow of venous blood. The antiseptic and fungicidal quality of indigo makes this oil good for the treatment of sprains, bruises and rheumatic pain. Bay harmonises with the throat chakra and also helps with earache, dizziness and balance. On an emotional level, Bay works through the indigo ray to release repressed emotions held in the hips and thighs as fat, by helping us express our true feelings through our words. Spiritually, Bay helps open the third eye chakra making connection to the unconscious mind especially through dreams – so use Bay essential oil in a sleepytime blue coloured pillow.

Therapeutic uses	Aromatherapy	Colour therapy
Physical	loss of appetite, anorexia nervosa, flatulence	red to stomach
	scanty periods – tonic to the reproductive system	red to pelvis
	tonsillitis, earache, viral infections	indigo to throat and head
	tonic to the liver	green to liver
	disperses blood in bruises, soothes inflammation and prevents scarring	indigo over problem area
Emotional	soothing but warming to the emotions	indigo to sacral centre, and blue to throat
Mental	sedative and mild narcotic effect, use in cases of hysteria or over-excitement	indigo to neck and shoulders
Spiritual	helps connect with your intuition and unconscious mind	indigo to the third eye

Precautions: Avoid during pregnancy, usually non-toxic and non-irritant.

Affirmations: With the blue ray of the laurel I openly communicate with my inner being. The orange ray increases my fertility and attracts abundance to me.

BENZOIN
Styrax benzoin
Healing colours/s: red and orange
Colour aroma treatment/s: colour bath, colour massage, perfume, room diffuser, spray mists, colour compresses, colour cooking, colour aroma lamps, colour inhalation
Chakra affinity: base
Life qualities: happiness, contentment, confidence, security, determination, perseverance

Colour signature: This viscous oil is very Yang in nature and is made from a resinous scented gum which is collected directly from this large tropical tree. Benzoin is usually sold dissolved in ethyl glycol or lexane. Crude benzoin is solid/brittle. The strong energising effect of Benzoin comes from its reddish or orange-brown colouring. The tree is large and has an aura of stability, and together with the colouring of the oil, reveals an affinity with the base chakra which it energises. By opening this chakra we are made aware that we have all the inner resources to deal with all life's challenges. Benzoin has also been reputed to create a feeling of euphoria, which helps buffer one against obstruction and emotional pain. The red ray of Benzoin warms and tones the heart by stimulating circulation and is excellent for the treatment of colds and chills. Its ability to relax muscle tissue makes it a useful oil for cracked and dry skin conditions and also gives us a more elastic and flexible approach to life. The leaves of the Styrax benzoin are pale green and citrus-like, so that the oil also reflects some yellow-green energy which gives it an antiseptic and astringent quality.

Therapeutic uses	Aromatherapy	Colour therapy
Physical	a warming relaxer which stimulates circulation and so aids arthritic and rheumatic conditions	red to soles of the feet
	opens the lungs allowing easier breathing	orange to chest
	strengthens the immune system – flu	orange to thymus and adrenals
	clears the skin and makes it glow	yellow to lungs
Emotional	eases and warms nervous tension and stress	yellow to solar-plexus
	gives confidence and helps emotional fatigue	
	warms the heart where there is disconnection from the emotions	orange to heart chakra
	encourages one to take life as it comes, helps let go of worries	orange to base chakra
Mental	calms the nerves and eases mental stress, makes the mind drowsy, freeing psychic states	colour breathing and visualisation
Spiritual	spiritually comforting, brings new hope where there has been alienation	red to base chakra
	grounding and promotes contentment	red to base chakra

Precautions: Use in moderation. Like the colour yellow, too much Benzoin can lead to headaches and nausea.

Affirmations: With the pink ray, my life is relaxed and I draw abundance to me. (Place a drop of oil directly on the pulse before saying the affirmation)

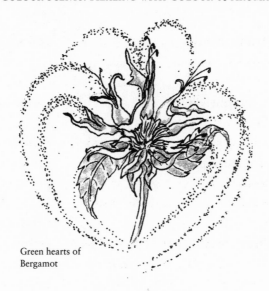

Green hearts of
Bergamot

BERGAMOT

CITRUS BERGAMIA

Healing colours/s: green and yellow
Colour aroma treatment/s: Colour compresses, colour breathing, spray
mists, solar charged water and tea, colour gargle, colour bath
Chakra affinity: sacral and solar-plexus
Life qualities: loving, joyous interchange, compassion, harmony,
centredness

Colour signature: Bergamot oil is made from the berries of a small tree, bearing small round fruit which ripen from green to yellow much like an orange. While most Bergamot oils have an affinity with the colour green, with ageing some oils turn brownish-olive revealing yellow and orange vibrations. So while Bergamot has a refreshing and balancing quality of green, its warm vibrations act as a general tonic leaving one feeling renewed and uplifted. The green energy within Bergamot makes it a healing and antiseptic oil which is useful to treatments of problems relating to the mouth and respiratory infections while its affinity with the heart chakra makes it excellent for alleviating shock and all types of stress. The purifying quality of yellow also ensures Bergamot is useful for the treatment of skin problems such as acne, boils, sores, eczema, spots and wounds and also has a positive effect on the digestive and genito-urinary and immune systems. The stronger yellow and even orange vibrations of some Bergamot oil helps develop our assertiveness and confidence, allowing us to improve our performance and creativity.

Therapeutic uses	Aromatherapy	Colour therapy
Physical	cooling and healing, use for skin problems, insect bites	yellow over affected area
	mouth infections, sore throat, tonsillitis	green over throat
	loss of appetite	orange over abdomen
	thrush, cystitis, leucorrhea	green over pelvic area
	gallstones, intestinal antiseptic	green over lower abdomen
	flu, infections, fever	green over chest
Emotional	good for anxiety and depression, and stress related conditions	yellow light irradiation to the whole body or solar-plexus
	soothing in highly emotional states	green light irradiation to whole body
	good for shock, hysteria	green light irradiation to whole body
Mental	refreshing and uplifting to the mind but also sedating	green to the soles of of the feet
Spiritual	sedating effect stills the conscious mind allowing us access to our intuition and higher mind	green over the crown chakra

Precautions: non-toxic (although photo-toxic if going into the sun), non-irritant.

Affirmations: I feel uplifted and refreshed as the yellow ray runs through my system. The green ray brings coolness and healing to my skin.

BIRCH

BETULA ALLEGHANIENSIS

Healing colours/s: yellow and violet
Colour aroma treatment/s: colour massage, spray mists and lotions, colour compresses, colour aromatic cooking, colour aroma lamps, room diffusers, perfumes, colour breathing,
Chakra affinity: solar-plexus and crown
Life qualities: centredness, quiet strength and knowing, peace, enlightenment

Colour signature: The yellow birch is a large woodland tree with branches which slope downwards and with serrated oval leaves. The long catkins bestow it with healing qualities of the two complementary colours of yellow and violet. Yellow is a purging and cleansing colour while violet also has a toning and purifying action. The sap has been used as a diuretic tea for skin preparations due to its astringent properties and in Scandinavia, young birch twigs are used to promote circulation in the sauna. The White Birch (Betula alba) which has silvery-white bark, has pain relieving properties commonly used in aspirin, and its white colour signature also gives it an affinity with the mind and head in general. The bark from the birch peels off in layers suggesting a healing quality of helping us shed unwanted baggage from the past.

Therapeutic uses	Aromatherapy	Colour therapy
Physical	purifies the blood, helping eliminate toxins through the skin	violet and yellow to whole body
	lymphatic cleanser, eliminates uric acid in the joints	yellow to affected areas, lymphatics
	dissolves stones in the kidney and bladder	violet to kidney and bladder
Emotional	helps you find your centre	yellow to solar-plexus, visualisation
	regaining dignity through self-value	violet to solar-plexus chakra

Mental	invigorating to the mind, dissolving fears	yellow to solar-plexus chakra
	bringing wisdom through linking to the higher mind	gold to crown chakra
Spiritual	brings release and deep healing through purging and cleansing the soul	violet to heart chakra
	transformative by raising the level of consciousness	violet to crown
	protection by raising the rate of vibration in the aura	violet to whole aura

Precautions: May irritate a sensitive skin. Use in maximum 1% dilution.

Affirmations: With the strength and protection of Birch, I am in tune with my inner self.

BLACK PEPPER
PIPER NIGRUM
Healing colours/s: red
Colour aroma treatment/s: colour compresses, foot baths using red towels, colour inhaler, colour breathing, colour candles
Chakra affinity: base
Life qualities: awareness, assertiveness, positivity, groundedness, security, action

Colour signature: The red colour signature of Black Pepper is extremely strengthening and stimulating opening our base chakra so that grounding earth energy can enter our system. Although it is known as black pepper, the berries turn from red to black as they mature giving Black Pepper a transformative quality. Thus pepper corns appear deep indigo when dried, but actually lock up the red energy inside them. The strong red vibration motivates us to find direction and to follow that path with endurance and fortitude. Its warming rosy-glow of energy develops inner security and helps us build up self-image and self-esteem and help develop assertiveness especially when we feel we are in a rut. When we have clarity of mind and develop intuitive vision, the qualities of the indigo ray, we have the tools with which we may come to know ourselves. The transformative quality of Black Pepper raises our consciousness from the physical to the spiritual realm.

Therapeutic uses	Aromatherapy	Colour therapy
Physical	strengthening to the whole body by aiding the formation of new blood cells	red to the liver
	builds immune system and a strong healthy body,	red to the soles of the feet
	warms and tones. Use for chilblains, anaemia, arthritis, muscular aches and pains, poor circulation, poor muscle tone, sprains, stiffness, chills	Light therapy to reflexes of feet.
	aids digestion of animal fats	red to the lower abdomen
Emotional	Instils a feeling of security, grounding and emotional stamina, warms the heart	Light therapy to base chakra
	promotes interaction when one is a non-participant, helps one act on a decision	red to base chakra
Mental	stimulating, and strengthening to the mind where mentally exhausted	indigo to the brow chakra
	motivation and perseverance where there is apathy	red to the base chakra

| *Spiritual* | Builds endurance to face life's ups and downs | red to the base chakra |
| | consciousness raising by opening the eye centre | indigo to third eye chakra |

Precautions: non-toxic, non-irritant, some people can be sensitive to this oil.

Affirmations: the red ray warms by body with vitality and strength and I am able to walk firmly on my chosen path in life.

CAJUPUT

MELALEUCA LEUCADENDRON

Healing colours/s: yellow, and violet

Colour aroma treatment/s: aroma spray mist, colour breathing, colour aroma massage (with caution), colour gargle

Chakra affinity: solar-plexus and crown

Life qualities: regeneration, transformation, relaxation, open but protected

Colour signature: This tall evergreen tree has thick pointed leaves and white flowers. The bark is white and spongy much like the lungs, and this makes Cajuput an ideal oil to use for the treatment of the respiratory tract and lung problems. The oil is a pale yellow-green and has a penetrating and camphorous aroma and its green tinge is derived from traces of copper found in the tree. The yellow ray in Cajuput makes it a warming and penetrating oil; it raises blood pressure without raising the heart beat. The complementary violet ray is also present, giving it antiseptic qualities. It is useful as an expectorant for gargles and as a freshening agent and for protection of the body from colds, flu and viral infections. Cajuput is mainly a physical oil, which has a drying and cleansing action on the skin. Cajeput is useful for pain relief and for treatment of any aches and pains in the head, ears, mouth. It is a well-known treatment for head lice and fleas and it is also useful for the treatment of problems of the genito-urinary system such as cystitis and urethritis. The Cajuput tree has the capacity for spontaneous re-growth after destruction, so its violet ray can help us recover and grow after trauma, by a process of transformation.

Therapeutic uses	Aromatherapy	Colour therapy
Physical	arthritis, aches and pains in the muscles, rheumatism – pain relief, oily skin, spots, insect bites, expels roundworm	yellow light over the affected area / yellow light, followed by violet over affect area. Also colour bandages
	asthma, bronchitis, catarrh, coughs, sinusitis, sore throat, laryngitis	yellow light over chest and throat in chronic cases (blue if acute)
	colds, flu, viral infections	violet light irradiation of whole body
Emotional	helps put the body and mind back into balance	violet over crown
Mental	clearing to the mind, stimulating	violet over crown
Spiritual	helps with spontaneous re-growth after emotional, mental or psychic attack.	violet over whole body

Precautions: Non-toxic, non-sensitising, use with care on a sensitive skin.

Affirmations: With the yellow ray, I am able to breathe more deeply and easily. The violet ray in Cajuput allows me to learn from every experience.

CAMPHOR
CINNAMOMUM CAMPHORA
Healing colours/s: red
Colour aroma treatment/s: Colour breathing, cold compresses, colour
room diffusers, hand and foot massage with light therapy
Chakra affinity: base
Life qualities: practicality, pioneering spirit, determination, focus,
clarity, purpose

Colour signature: Camphor is a large hardy evergreen tree, which grows
very tall. Its sturdy nature and strong earth connection give Camphor the
capacity to energise the base chakra, stimulating vital energy through the
body. The ancients believed camphor could give the body life after death
and so they used it as one of the main ingredients of embalming.
Camphor has a crystalline formation which is found in all parts of the tree
and its structure gives it the ability to amplify energy. The crystalline structure gives it an affinity with the pineal gland and third eye chakra, enabling
it to heighten self-awareness and giving us the ability to take decisive action
through clarity of mind. Camphor's red energy gives us motivation, and
lifts one out of a depression while encouraging us to display the qualities
of leadership. On the physical side it warms the body and stiff muscles,
and raises low blood pressure. It clears congestion throughout the body,
by moving blood and red energy through the system.

Therapeutic uses	Aromatherapy	Colour therapy
Physical	stimulates the heart raising blood pressure. Warms stiff muscles, rheumatism, aches and pains	red over affected area, but not the heart
	Works on urinary system and sexual organs	red light over kidneys or pelvis

Emotional	Although it is primary stimulating, this oil balances the emotions through grounding and opening the base chakra	red light to base chakra
	motivation, stamina and determination to get things done	red light to base chakra
Mental	Calms nervous energy by building up strength of mind and determination	red light through solar-plexus foot reflex
Spiritual	helps grounding and putting creative ideas into practice awakening us to life so we become conscious of every minute	red light on base chakra red colour breathing and meditation

Precautions: Avoid during pregnancy. Use in moderation, avoid in cases of epilepsy or convulsions. White camphor is less toxic than yellow or brown.

Affirmations: The red ray instils me with strength and determination.

CARAWAY
CARUM CARVI
Healing colours/s: orange/golden yellow/pink
Colour aroma treatment/s: colour aroma diffusers, colour candles, colour aromatic cooking, colour aroma bath, colour compress
Chakra affinity: sacral, solar-plexus and heart
Life qualities: Adds spice to life, radiant health, inner glow

Colour signature: The curved brown seeds of this herb also contain the pink energy of the flowers, making the oil an uplifting but gentle tonic. The seeds are full of sunlight and the natural affinity they have to the colour yellow energises the solar-plexus and acts as a blood cleanser and tonic to the liver. The gold and pink energy work in harmony to boost one's self-image so that one can accept oneself with love. Caraway is reputed to be a good tissue regenerator as the pink ray stimulates circulation so that oxygen is carried around the body. This is why, in ancient Greece young girls were given Caraway to bring colour to pale complexions. On a more subtle level, universal love is allowed to flow through the open solar-plexus and heart chakras so that we become more nurturing and caring of others. A strong solar-plexus provides strength and protection in times when the heart is troubled or when one is in a difficult emotional relationship.

Therapeutic uses	Aromatherapy	Colour therapy
Physical	stimulates circulation, regenerates tissue	orange to soles of feet
	a good general tonic	orange to whole body
	stimulates appetite and digestion	orange to stomach area
	helps lung and throat problems	orange to chest
	increases milk in nursing mothers	orange to chest area
Emotional	warming to the emotions	orange to sacral chakra
	helps release worries from the past	orange to sacral chakra
	tonic to the nerves, when suffering emotional strain	orange to solar-plexus
Mental	good for mental fatigue and strain	orange to whole body, colour breathing
	replenishes energy	orange to soles of feet
	brings wisdom into your affairs	colour breathing and meditation
Spiritual	Guards against loss of loved ones	orange/pink candles, meditation
	strengthens and re-charges aura	orange to whole body

Precautions: May irritate some sensitive skins

Affirmations: Caraway boosts my whole system, filling me with vitality and energy.

CARDAMOM
ELETTARIA CARDAMOMUM
Healing colours/s: orange, golden-yellow
Colour aroma treatment/s: colour breathing, colour aroma room diffuser, solar-charged drink, colour massage, colour aromatic cooking
Chakra affinity: sacral, solar-plexus and throat
Life qualities: focus, enthusiasm, empowerment, purpose, creativity

Colour signature: This is a leafy stemmed shrub with long pale yellow flowers with mauve tips. The oblong grey fruits contain seeds which are gathered just before they are ripe. On the physical level the cardamom operates on the orange and yellow ray and is an invigorating oil. The orange ray Cardamom contains is a tonic which increases sexual desire. The yellow ray aspect makes it useful for the treatment of digestive problems especially of nervous origin, as a carmative, stomachic and laxative. The yellow ray works on the nervous system, so that it relaxes one and so releasing PMS headaches and irritability. The yellow energy also helps strengthen the mind and allows self-development and expansion of one's view of life. It also lets us loosen up emotionally. The violet ray also reflected in Cardamom helps clear the head especially when we are confused or muddled, enabling us to see our way more clearly.

Therapeutic uses	Aromatherapy	Colour therapy
Physical	colic, cramp, dyspepsia, flatulence, griping pains, heartburn, vomiting, indigestion	yellow over liver
	invigorating, use for low sexual drive	orange over pelvis
	warms the body, eases coughs	orange over chest

Emotional	PMS related problems marked by headaches and irritability	blue over solar-plexus chakra
	warming to the emotions promotes creativity and self-expression	orange over sacral chakra
Mental	mental fatigue and weakness due to nervous strain	yellow over solar-plexus
	clarifying and aids concentration	yellow to crown chakra
Spiritual	opens the hara so one's own radiance can shine through	gold to hara centre, visualisation

Precautions: non-toxic, non-irritant, non-sensitising

Affirmations: The yellow ray in Cardamom calms my nerves bringing me peace and tranquillity. The orange ray warms my body and gives me vitality and energy.

CARROT SEED
DAUCUS CAROTA
Healing colours/s: orange, golden-yellow and violet
Colour aroma treatment/s: colour baths, colour massage, spray mists, colour compresses, colour aromatic cooking, colour aroma lamps, room diffusers, perfumes, colour breathing
Chakra affinity: solar-plexus, crown
Life qualities: Joy, inner-strength, self-expression, expansion

Colour signature: The oil of Carrot Seed is a beautiful amber liquid giving Carrot Seed its strong orange and golden-yellow colour signature. The flowers of the carrot plant are purple and so the oil contains both yellow and purple energy. These complementary colours work together, the yellow acting as a tonic to body and mind, the violet bringing about changes and transformation at a deeper level. Both yellow and violet have a cleansing action. The yellow cleanses the gall-bladder and liver helping to release repressed emotions of jealousy, resentment and greed while the violet releases the mental and emotional pain caused by these emotions. Carrot Seed is highly nutritious making it useful in the treatment of anorexia. The orange ray stimulates the appetite while the violet ray balances metabolism and the psyche, releasing fears and phobias related to eating.

Therapeutic uses	Aromatherapy	Colour therapy
Physical	tonic to reproductive and digestive system	orange to stomach and lower abdomen
	muscle relaxant – promotes menstruation	orange to pelvis
	tonic to gall-bladder and liver	orange to liver
	stimulates appetite, nutritious, so good for treatment of anorexia	orange to stomach / violet to crown
Emotional	nourishing to the emotions	orange to solar-plexus chakra
	self-expression in sexual and emotional relationships	orange to sacral chakra
	provides stamina and fortitude in the face of hardship	yellow to solar-plexus
Mental	relieves stress and mental exhaustion	gold to crown
	cleansing effect on the mind, driving out destructive thoughts	gold and violet to solar-plexus and crown
Spiritual	releases deep-seated pain from the causal plane (from previous lives)	violet to crown
	brings joy into your life	orange to whole body, colour breathing

Precautions: Avoid during pregnancy.

Affirmations: Carrot Seed frees the spirit and brings joy into my life.

CEDARWOOD
JUNIPERUS VIRGINIANA
Healing colours/s: red, orange and yellow
Colour aroma treatment/s: colour bath, colour massage, perfume, room diffuser, spray mists, colour compresses, colour cooking, colour aroma lamps
Chakra affinity: base, sacral and solar-plexus
Life qualities: grounding, strengthening, focus, purposeful action, dignity

Colour signature: This pyramid shaped evergreen tree grows to majestic proportions and is a tower of strength pointing to the sky. The Semitic word for 'Cedar' means power of spiritual strength and because of these enduring qualities the wood was used for embalming in ancient times. The oil gives Cedarwood its colour signature being yellow, orange or deep amber, all of which activate the lower chakras. It is particularly good for alleviating chronic conditions as the energy blocks created by repressed emotions are dissolved as deep-seated fears and worries are released. The energising nature of the tree allows one to be a pillar of strength, helping us find our true path in life and our life's purpose. The centring and releasing action of the energy allows connection to the higher mind and so the vibrations released from Cedarwood are a good meditation aid.

Therapeutic uses	Aromatherapy	Colour therapy
Physical	expectorant, dries out 'phlegm'	orange to chest
	helps arthritis and rheumatism	red to lower pelvis and kidneys
	helps genito-urinary problems	orange to bladder and kidneys and lower pelvis

Emotional	comforting to the heart giving fortitude in times of hardship	orange to sacral chakra
	improves self-image, self-esteem	yellow to solar-plexus
	counteracts shyness and promotes assertiveness	orange to solar-plexus, affirmations
Mental	boosts mental faculties where there is mental strain	red to base chakra
	releases obsessions, paranoia by promoting inner security	red to base chakra, gemstone healing
	boosts the nervous system	orange to sacral chakra
	spiritual strength and determination	colour breathing and visualisation
Spiritual	aid to meditation by grounding and inner focus	colour meditation

Precautions: Avoid during pregnancy. May irritate the skin.

Affirmations: With the warming magnetic rays in Cedarwood, I can rely on my inner strength to face any challenges which come my way.

CELERY
APIUM GRAVEOLENS
Healing colours/s: Yellow and green
Colour aroma treatment/s: spray mists, colour compresses, colour aromatic cooking, colour aroma lamps, room diffusers, perfumes, colour breathing
Chakra affinity: sacral, solar-plexus, heart
Life qualities: Gentleness with strength, freshness, brightness, prosperity

Colour signature: This delicate plant has an erect stalk, shiny pinnate leaves and umbrellas of white flowers. Celery is best known as a vegetable rather than a medicinal herb, but it contains a balance of light energy, making it very useful for healing at many levels. Although the paleness of the plant indicates a light colour signature, the essential oil which is made from the small seeds has a yellow or orange colouring, showing that it also carries strong magnetic energy. Indeed, celery oil is both a tonic and a sedative, indicating that this oil works on several levels simultaneously. The green ray soothes, cools and cleanses, while the warming rays have regenerative and restorative properties. Its slightly intoxicating and euphoric action, is restorative to a tired mind as it frees up thoughts, and helps balance the psyche especially where there is over attention to detail and trivialities.

Therapeutic uses	Aromatherapy	Colour therapy
Physical	cools fevers and reduces blood pressure	green over heart
	cleanses the skin through the elimination of toxins from the blood – good for reducing water retention	yellow over liver
	restores libido and is useful for a range of menstrual problems	orange of lower body
	cleanses liver and good for indigestion	green over liver
Emotional	brings sexual satisfaction and pleasure through discrimination and self-esteem	orange to lower body
	opens the heart, allowing freshness and brightness and prosperity to enter	green to heart chakra
Mental	lifts mental depression	orange to whole body
	tonic to the tired mind	orange to whole body or feet

| *Spiritual* | Balances the psyche – combines flexibility and softness with strength | green to heart chakra |
| | grounding, while giving lightness of spirit | colour breathing and meditation |

Precautions: Avoid during pregnancy.

Affirmations: With the cleansing and balancing rays in Celery, I am filled with lightness and feel fresh and renewed.

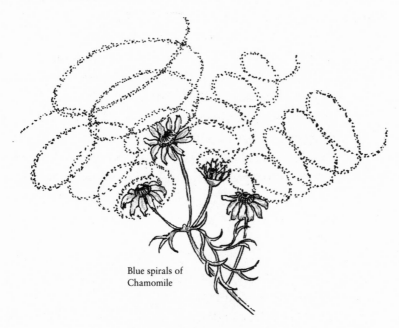

Blue spirals of
Chamomile

CHAMOMILE (GERMAN)
MATRICARIA CHAMOMILLA
Healing colours/s: blue
Colour aroma treatment/s: colour baths, colour massage, spray mists, solarised tea and water, colour compresses, skin preparations, colour sleepy-time pillow
Chakra affinity: throat
Life properties: patience, calmness, peace, relaxation, healing

Colour signature: This pretty herb has feathery leaves with small white flowers with a yellow centre and is smaller than Roman chamomile. German chamomile has the affinity with the blue vibration and takes its colour signature from the Azulene which becomes apparent in the essential oil. This chamomile oil is a deeper blue than the Roman variety, and it contains powerful anti-inflammatory qualities. The ancient Egyptians used Chamomile to treat nervous complaints and to soothe and cool many ailments including skin care. The blue ray is reflected in the delicate quality of the plant and its mild and gentle healing action can be used with safety on children, the weak and the elderly. Blue is calming and relaxing to the emotions and mind, and this makes Chamomile excellent for treating anxiety, tension, anger and fear through communication and expression through the throat chakra. It sedates the mind, and promotes sleep.

Therapeutic uses	Aromatherapy	Colour therapy
Physical	generally cooling and healing, use in cases of nervous dyspepsia, nervous bowel	indigo to solar-plexus
	tension headaches, sleeplessness menstrual problems	indigo to back of head indigo to lower abdomen
	dermatitis, eczema, psoriasis, burns	indigo to affected area
Emotional	worry, tension, nervousness, releases anger and fear apprehension, timidity	indigo to third eye chakra
Mental	nervous tension, headaches, relaxes the mind calming and understanding, helps one connect with one's intuition	indigo to third eye
Spiritual	brings peace and patience	indigo to third eye

Precautions: non-toxic, non-irritant, non-sensitising

Affirmations: The deep blue of chamomile relieves my tension and lets me relax. My pain leaves me as I breathe in the deep blue vibration. I am calm and at peace.

CHAMOMILE (ROMAN)
ANTHEMIS NOBILIS
Healing colours/s: blue
Colour aroma treatment/s: colour bath, colour massage, solarised lotions and skin preparations, colour aroma lamps, spray mists
Chakra affinity: throat
Life qualities: serenity, peace, intuition, calmness, co-operation, knowledge, spirituality

Colour signature: This small spreading or creeping herb has feathery leaves and white daisy-like flowers and has a sharp apple-like scent. The oil yields a pale blue liquid with a warm, sweet herbaceous scent. Chamomile has an affinity with the colour blue, which is particularly soothing, cooling, calming and healing. Its blue signature brings softness, gentleness and is especially good for dispelling anger, frustration, irritation or hysteria. The oil is useful for any hot condition like fevers, inflammations, sunstroke or burns. As the blue vibrations relax the emotions and mind, Roman Chamomile is good for the treatment of most painful conditions and stress. The pain-relieving qualities of blue extend to the subtle bodies, and the calming vibrations of this oil make it excellent for all kinds of emotional and stressful conditions, especially in times of trauma or when someone feels they cannot cope with life.

Therapeutic uses	Aromatherapy	Colour therapy
Physical	soothes aches and pains, use for painful muscles and joints, arthritis	blue over affected and followed by orange
	neuralgia, rheumatism, sprains	blue over feet, legs
	menopausal problems	blue to pituitary gland
	anti-inflammatory, gentle and soothes hot dry skin, sunburn and other skin conditions.	blue to affected area
	headaches, nervous tension, stress, migraine	blue to crown
Emotional	anxiety, worry, hysteria, weepiness, emotional violence, loneliness, grief, anger, withdrawal of emotions, self-blame	blue to the throat and sacral area
Mental	relaxing the mind, sleep inducing	blue to whole body
Spiritual	depression, insomnia, nervous exhaustion, amnesia,	blue to crown chakra
	inner peace and stillness	blue to whole body

Precautions: non-toxic, non-irritant, non-sensitising

Affirmations: With the blue ray in Roman chamomile I am at peace with myself and the world. The blue ray brings me relief from pain, so that I can learn the lesson it brings me.

CLOVE

EUGENIA CARYOPHYLLATA

Healing colours/s: indigo

Colour aroma treatment/s: room diffusers, colour aroma lamps, spray mists, local colour compresses, perfumes, solar charged food and water

Chakra affinity: third eye

Life qualities: focus, vision, idealism, knowledge, insight

Colour signature: The clove is well known in cooking and the essential oil takes its colour signature from the dark blue-black seed pods from this evergreen tree. The strong indigo ray reflected in clove gives it pain relieving properties especially for areas around the face. It can be used to ease toothache and mouth ulcers, and relieve tension headaches. The disinfectant qualities make Clove oil excellent for helping the body resist germs, while its red vibration as a spice works on the digestive system, helping cure diarrhoea, intestinal spasm, dyspepsia and bad breath caused by an upset stomach. Indigo energy flushes out the kidneys and spleen, the main organs which extract life force energy or prana from the bloodstream. The aroma and colour energy in clove makes it pervasive and stimulating to the mind, strengthening memory and encouraging positive thoughts. It can release emotional problems by bringing them into focus, so assisting self-awareness with understanding.

Therapeutic uses	Aromatherapy	Colour therapy
Physical	pain relief during childbirth	indigo on soles of feet or lower back
	tonic to kidneys, stomach, spleen	Indigo over kidneys, stomach
	intestinal spasm and parasites, dyspepsia, diarrhoea	indigo over lower abdomen
	rheumatism, arthritis	indigo over soles of feet and joints
	general pain relief, mouth sores and ulcers	indigo light over painful area

Emotional	releases the emotions through inner knowledge, aids creative expression of feelings, lifts lethargy and feeling weakness	indigo over third eye chakra
Mental	stimulating when lethargic or disinterested, strengthens memory and helps focus	indigo over third eye chakra
Spiritual	brings happiness and contentment through self-awareness, cleanses the aura	indigo over third eye

Precautions: Use with caution on localised areas only. Can cause skin irritation.

Affirmations: With the Indigo ray in Clove Bud I think positive and happy thoughts.
Clove and the Indigo ray brings calmness, coolness and quiet into my system.

CINNAMON

CINNAMOMUM ZEYLANICUM

Healing colours/s: orange and yellow, indigo
Colour aroma treatment/s: spray mists, colour compresses, colour aromatic cooking, colour aroma lamps, room diffusers, perfumes, colour breathing,
Chakra affinity: sacral, solar-plexus
Life qualities: liberty, justice, benevolence, creativity, energy, sensuality

Colour signature: This exotic rust-coloured evergreen tree has thick bark with green-orange speckled shoots. The leaves are green and leathery and its small white flowers appear throughout the year. The tree has bluish berries. The strong orange-yellow colour signature is found in the oil which is made from the familiar brown quills which are rolled up inside one another. The orange ray peels off the layers of bark drawing one out where one is too introverted and making one more direct and truthful in one's dealings with others. The orange ray lifts depression and the golden ray helps bring joy and happiness into your life. The complementary deep blue colouring of the berries also has an underlying influence, acting as a sedative and instilling one with the qualities of fair-play, loyalty and trust.

Therapeutic uses	Aromatherapy	Colour therapy
Physical	stimulates the glandular system when one feels weak and exhausted	orange to the soles of the feet and pituitary gland
	raises body temperature, stimulates circulation or a sluggish digestion	orange to whole body
	eases muscular spasms	orange to affected area
	eases breathing by expanding the chest	orange to chest
	eases childbirth	orange colour breathing or light to whole body
Emotional	warming and strengthening, freeing action, putting one in touch with ones body and sensuality	orange to whole body orange to sacral chakra
	picks one up after nervous exhaustion	orange to whole body, feet
Mental	lifts depression, energiser	orange to whole body, affirmations
	gives one strength of purpose	orange visualisation, gemstone healing
	links to ones creativity in a practical way	orange to whole body or sacral chakra
Spiritual	brings alertness and focus	indigo to brow chakra
	promotes higher ideals	indigo to brow centre

Precautions: Can cause severe skin reactions and convulsions. Use in max 1% dilution.

Affirmations: With the orange ray in Cinnamon I have a realistic attitude whereby I can take direct action.

CITRONELLA
CYMBOPOGON NARDUS
Healing colours/s: yellow
Colour aroma treatment/s: colour baths, household and body spray mists, aromatic colour candles, colour cooking, colour aroma lamps, room diffusers, insect repellents
Chakra affinity: solar-plexus
Life qualities: clear thinking, alert, versatile, wise, assertive, logical

Colour signature: Citronella is a tall aromatic grass with a yellow stem and leaves. The oil has a strong colour signature and is a good overall tonic. The citronella grass grows upright in large clumps and while being flexible, it is well-grounded. The yellow ray of Citronella has an affinity with the mind, clearing the head and assisting concentration. It promotes general alertness and lifts headaches and migraines. Its healing qualities thus bring security and strength while allowing openness of mind attracting new inspiration. Citronella is a well-known insect deterrent, and this protective quality also wards off harmful vibrations of mischievous spirits and devas from rooms around the house.

Therapeutic uses	Aromatherapy	Colour therapy
Physical	tones the digestive and reproductive systems	yellow to stomach and reproductive organs
	eases rheumatic aches and pains	yellow to soles of the feet
	deodorant, and anti-insect control	candles, spray mists, room diffusers

138

Emotional	strengthens and uplifts the emotions when emotionally drained	yellow to heart chakra
	Helps one build self-confidence and find personal power	yellow to solar-plexus chakra
	helps communication with others by keeping an open mind	gold to solar-plexus, colour breathing
Mental	clears and lifts depression	yellow to solar-plexus
	aids memory and concentration and improves general alertness	yellow to solar-plexus or soles of feet
Spiritual	gives direction and wisdom through inspiration and inner connection	gold to crown chakra
	wards off harmful vibrations and psychic attack	gold visualisation, aromatic candles, room diffuser

Precautions: Avoid during pregnancy. May irritate a sensitive skin.

Affirmations: With the yellow ray in Citronella I value myself and can express my deep feelings.

CLARY SAGE
SALVIA SCLAREA
Healing colours/s: magenta and violet
Colour aroma treatment/s: colour aroma lamps, colour massage, colour aroma baths, colour breathing, spray mists, perfumes, solar charged water
Chakra affinity: crown and base
Life qualities: tranquillity, vitality, balance, relaxation, strength in stillness

Colour signature: Clary sage is a herb with large hairy leaves which are green with a hint of purple, and small blue mauve flowers. The oil is colourless or a pale yellow green with a nutty herbaceous aroma. Clary sage is cooling and soothing, and the mucilage from the seeds is used for treating tumours. It has a cleansing action on the digestive system, which alleviates cramps, flatulence and dyspepsia. The violet ray activates the central nervous system, making Clary Sage a good nerve tonic while the grounding red vibration energises the kidneys, flushing them through thus strengthening the flow of energy in the body. Clary Sage is therefore good for nervous exhaustion and the treatment of stress. The purple ray balances and harmonises the crown chakra, exerting a transformative action on the psyche. It is useful for treating problems such as phobias, obsession, rage, and fear. Clary Sage also reflects the transformative quality of violet which encourages a mature attitude to life and the ability to see life in perspective. The sedative effects of its colour frequency together with its grounding ability help release unfounded fears and emotional breakdown by building self-confidence and security through the energy in the kidneys.

Therapeutic uses	Aromatherapy	Colour therapy
Physical	all inflamed conditions, ulcers, high blood pressure and pains	violet on soles of the feet
	throat infections, whooping cough, asthma,	violet to throat
	cramp, dyspepsia, flatulence, labour pains	violet over abdomen violet over pelvis and lower back
Emotional	releasing of guilt and fears through transformation of energy	violet over crown chakra
	makes one sleepy and amorous	magenta to base chakra
	builds inner strength and confidence	violet over base and crown

Mental	depression, migraine, nervous tension and stress	violet over crown chakra
	releases fears of the mind, paranoia, obsession and delusions	violet over the crown chakra
Spiritual	promotes humility and self-sacrifice and the giving of unconditional love	magenta over base, violet over crown

Precautions: non-toxic, non-irritant, non-sensitising, avoid during pregnancy.

Affirmations: With the violet ray, all my tensions and worries leave me.

CORIANDER

Coriandrum sativum

Healing colours/s: yellow, green and pink
Colour aroma treatment/s: colour baths, colour massage, spray mists and lotions, colour compresses, colour aromatic cooking, colour aroma lamps, room diffusers, perfumes, colour breathing
Chakra affinity: solar-plexus and heart
Life qualities: optimism, enthusiasm, creativity, co-operation, kindness

Colour signature: This strongly aromatic herb has feathery leaves and pinkish white flowers. The crushed seeds, from which the oil is made are brownish-green and yield a colourless liquid with a woody-spicy aroma. Coriander has a mixture of notes. The strength of the aroma gives coriander a middle note, while the pink ray gives it a top note. Pink is gently warming to the emotions, and as it contains white light, it helps free blocks allowing white light energy to flow through the subtle bodies, refreshing and renewing the life-force within the individual. The yellow/green rays work on a more physical level, toning and cleansing and giving coriander an uplifting and refreshing quality. The affinity of this oil with the digestive system together with the lightness of the vibrations have made it renowned for healing childhood problems such as diarrhoea, griping pains, flatulence and colic.

Therapeutic uses	Aromatherapy	Colour therapy
Physical	gently warms the body without raising the pulse, good for muscle spasms, flu, lung problems	yellow to feet or whole body
	clears toxins from the body by stimulating the spleen	yellow to spleen
	warms the stomach, aids digestion	yellow to stomach
Emotional	helps one release and cleanse repressed emotions by expressing oneself joyously and creatively	yellow to solar-plexus
	opens the heart by sharing problems	green to heart and throat
Mental	lifts depression and anxiety	yellow to crown chakra
	uplifting and refreshing to the mind	green to crown chakra
	aids memory and promotes optimism	yellow to crown chakra
Spiritual	renews the flow of life force energy by activating the spleen	gold or white colour breathing
	helps you 'go with the flow'	gold to solar-plexus, colour breathing

Precautions: Stupefying in large doses.

Affirmations: With Coriander, I become a channel for life-force energy which flows through me connecting me to the cosmic forces.

CUMIN

CUMINUM CYMINUM

Healing colours/s: yellow and pink
Colour aroma treatment/s: spray mists, colour compresses, colour aromatic cooking, colour aroma lamps, room diffusers, perfumes, colour breathing
Chakra affinity: solar-plexus and heart
Life qualities: exchange, sharing, intimacy, warmth, positivity

Colour signature: The oil is made from distillation of the ripe seeds of this small delicate herb. The plant has a slender appearance with dark green feathery leaves and small pink or white flowers which change to the fruits yielding the yellow seeds. The pale yellow colouring of the oil reveals its medicinal use on the physical body, and its affinity with the digestion and nervous system. The colour yellow also helps regulate the metabolic processes. The pinky colouring of the flowers gives the oil a top note which acts upon the subtle bodies to balance the mind and psychological states and open the heart to healing. Cumin is known to have a beneficial action on the reproductive system of both men and women and it is through the pink ray which helps open our heart and soul to others that reinforces this ability to share and care in a sexual relationship. The Hindus think of Cumin as a symbol of fidelity, and it is this undercurrent of compassion and intimacy in a relationship which gives the oil these therapeutic characteristics.

Therapeutic uses	Aromatherapy	Colour therapy
Physical	beneficial to the liver, elimination of toxins and congestion in the body	yellow to liver
	stimulates the digestive system	yellow to stomach area
	aphrodisiac	yellow and pink to pelvis and hips
	stimulates circulation	yellow to soles of the feet

Emotional	frees emotions and allows sexual intimacy	yellow to solar-plexus
	exchange while keeping personal power intact	yellow to solar-plexus
Mental	aids communication and stimulates the mind gives a positive outlook	yellow to the crown
	helps link to one's higher mind through an open heart	pink to the heart chakra
Spiritual	celebration of who we are	gold to the heart chakra
	joyous love for the world	gold to the heart chakra

Precautions: Avoid during pregnancy, can irritate the skin. The aroma can be overpowering.

Affirmations: With the yellow energy in Cumin, I cleanse myself of all congestion in the body, emotions and mind.

CYPRESS
Cupressus sempervirens
Healing colours/s: blue and orange
Colour aroma treatment/s: colour massage, colour baths, colour aroma lamps, colour breathing, colour compresses, colour poultices
Chakra affinity: throat and sacral
Life qualities: generosity, inner peace, structure, straightforwardness

Colour signature: This tall evergreen tree has a conical shape, and bears small flowers with round brown-grey nuts and reddish-yellow wood. Cypress trees are a common sight in gardens and cemeteries in Mediterranean countries. Cypress is a solitary and quiet tree which appears to stand guard and once cut it never grows again. These trees are thought to have strong protective qualities and cleanse negative vibrations from grave-yards and churches. The oil is distilled from the twigs, needles and cones, but its blue colour vibration comes mainly from its connection with the throat chakra and its sympathetic action on the respiratory system. The quiet and dignified Cypress tree makes its oil excellent for the treatment of over-talkative people who like to gossip. It is also good in cases where any sort of excess is present. Its strength and wisdom comes from the orange ray also found in the oil, but sensitivity and compassion from the blue. The blue vibration in Cypress has a constricting effect on veins and body fluids, which is helpful for treating varicose veins and haemorrhoids.

Therapeutic uses	Aromatherapy	Colour therapy
Physical	reduces excessive flow of fluids, nose bleeds, heavy menstruation, sweating, incontinence, heavy sweating	blue to lower back or throat
	lung problems, whooping cough, flu, asthma, bronchitis	blue over chest
	balancing action on the skin through limiting sweating	blue to soles of feet
Emotional	soothes anger, prevents withdrawal from life, grief, regrets, breakdown, mood swings	blue to throat chakra
	learning to trust	blue to throat chakra
Mental	forgetfulness, depression, amnesia due to fear	blue to crown and solar-plexus
Spiritual	cleanses spirit and removes psychic blocks brings inner peace and purity of heart	blue light irradiation to whole body

Precautions: non-toxic, non-irritant, non-sensitising, apply to affected areas only and not for general massage. Avoid in pregnancy.

Affirmations: Cypress helps me keep my integrity in what I say and do. With the orange ray in Cypress I can release my fears and express myself.

DILL
Anethum graveolens
Healing colours/s: yellow
Colour aroma treatment/s: colour baths, colour massage, colour compresses, colour aromatic cooking, colour aroma lamps, room diffusers, perfumes, colour breathing,
Chakra affinity: solar-plexus
Life qualities: Self-confidence, free thinking, good judgement, magical

Colour signature: The oil of Dill is distilled from the fruit or seed of this dark green feathery-leafed herb. The compressed flat fruits develop from multiple heads of small yellow flowers yielding a colourless to pale yellow oil with a strong warm spicy aroma. Historically, Dill was considered a magical herb, and used by sorcerers and magicians for spell-casting and for the protection of houses against evil spirits. Although the plant looks fragile, it contains a strong yellow vibration which is particular resonant with the digestive system. Its use as a culinary herb has been known since ancient times. When baked in bread it soothes the digestion especially in the old or young. The spreading tops of yellow flowers reveal a freeing action on the mind and emotions, allowing free thinking and promoting self-confidence. Dill has a calming action on both body and mind by feeding the nervous system and by uplifting the spirits creating space to enjoy new experiences and ideas.

Therapeutic uses	Aromatherapy	Colour therapy
Physical	soothing to the digestion, use for flatulence and constipation	yellow over stomach area
	eases cramps	yellow to affected area
	eases childbirth and promotes flow of mother's milk	yellow deep breathing and visualisations inhalation
Emotional	builds confidence and recognition of inner strength	yellow to solar-plexus chakra
	releases worry and fear	yellow to solar-plexus
	helps you cope with shock and crises	yellow to solar-plexus and violet to crown
Mental	soporific action on the mind, freeing it from worry and cares	yellow to soles of the feet
	eases headaches and good for insomnia	yellow to temples or back of head
Spiritual	opens the crown chakra by freeing the lower mind from fears and restrictive patterns	gold to crown
	promotes receptivity to other worlds	gold to crown and solar-plexus

Precautions: Avoid during pregnancy.

Affirmations: With the yellow ray in Dill I use my inner strength to cope with the challenges I am now facing.

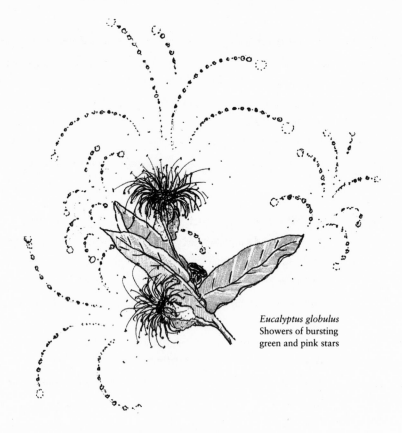

Eucalyptus globulus
Showers of bursting
green and pink stars

EUCALYPTUS

EUCALYPTUS GLOBULUS

Healing colours/s: green and pink (some varieties blue)
Colour aroma treatment/s: colour inhaler, colour breathing, colour
aroma lamp, room spray mist, solar-charged deodorant
Chakra affinity: heart
Life qualities: vitality, harmony, love, receptivity, contentment, balance

Colour signature: Eucalyptus is a beautiful tall evergreen tree native to Australia. Mature trees have narrow yellowish leaves and creamy white flowers. Peppermint Eucalyptus has young leaves which are blue and heart-shaped, while the lemon-scented variety has attractive grey, cream and pinky coloured bark. Many plants which have an affinity with the green ray have heart-shaped leaves and this connection with the heart chakra brings emotional freedom, contentment and wholeness, where there was a feeling of emptiness. The aroma of Eucalyptus promotes deep breathing while the green expands and relaxes the chest and lungs making it a useful oil in the relief of respiratory complaints. Eucalyptus also lowers temperature and reduces painful headaches and migraines. It has a similar effect on the emotions, cooling and calming in cases of over-excitement, moodiness or addictive behaviour.

Therapeutic uses	Aromatherapy	Colour therapy
Physical	sore throat, soothes respiratory tract, clears mucus	green over chest and neck
	clears head of hay fever, colds, infections	green over chest and throat
	decongests liver, dissolves gallstones, helps control diabetes	green over liver
	muscular aches and pains	green on feet
Emotional	cools and comforts, dissolves bitterness and resentment	green over heart chakra
	helps get rid of addictions, guilt and self-blame	green over heart chakra
Mental	lifts depression, clears head, aids concentration, strengthens nerves	green over crown
Spiritual	clears a path for past life recall, regenerative by opening the heart to universal love	green candle and oil for meditation and relaxation

Precautions: non-toxic, avoid in cases of high blood pressure, epilepsy. Use in moderation.

Affirmations: Eucalyptus clears my lungs, throat and head.
The green energy in Eucalyptus allows me to love those whom I envy, am jealous of, resent or hate.

FENNEL

FOENICULUM VULGARE

Healing colours/s: yellow
Colour aroma treatment/s: colour baths, colour massage, spray mists and lotions, colour aromatic cooking, colour aroma lamps, perfumes, colour breathing,
Chakra affinity: solar-plexus, heart
Life qualities: confidence, assertiveness, enlightenment

Colour signature: This tall herb has feathery leaves and golden yellow flowers which are very attractive to bees. The oil is a pale yellow made from the crushed seeds and yields a sweet anise-like scent. In ancient times, it was believed that Fennel was imbued with the power to bring courage, strength and longevity. Although fennel has a flimsy appearance, its strength comes from the profusion and vigorous growth of this herb together with its golden-yellow colour signature. The vibrations from this sea of softness bring us strength and determination to overcome life's challenges, while remaining flexible and sensitive to the feelings of others. Fennel is probably best known for its use in cooking and as a slimming aid. The yellow energy has a diuretic action, cleansing toxins from the body by clearing obstructions in the liver and gall-bladder. On a psychological level, yellow promotes confidence and assertiveness, both of which are necessary when trying to treat eating disorders.

Therapeutic uses	Aromatherapy	Colour therapy
Physical	strengthens the eyes	green to eye reflexes on feet
	expectorant action for asthma, bronchitis and lung congestion	yellow to the chest
	cleanses liver and gall-bladder	green to the liver and gall-bladder
	cleanses and tones an oily skin, helps remove cellulite and water retention	yellow colour breathing, yellow to whole body

Emotional	renews our interest in life	yellow to the solar-plexus
	regulates hormones, bringing balance	yellow to the pituitary gland
	for nurturing self-love and respect, helping us value ourselves	green to the heart chakra
Mental	releases creative block	yellow to the crown chakra
	brings fortitude to pursue our chosen path in life	yellow to the base chakra
	promotes clear thinking	yellow to the crown chakra
Spiritual	opens us to our own inner wisdom	gold to the crown chakra
	enlightenment and protection through strength	gold to whole aura, meditation

Precautions: Avoid during pregnancy and cases of epilepsy. Toxic in large doses.

Affirmations: With the protection of Fennel, I regain my self-confidence and spirit of adventure.

FIR

Abies balsamea
Healing colours/s: green
Colour aroma treatment/s: colour baths, colour massage, spray mists, colour compresses, colour aroma lamps, room diffusers and inhalation, perfumes, colour breathing
Chakra affinity: heart
Life qualities: freedom, liberation, expansion, openness

Colour signature: There are many species of these evergreens around the world. Abies balsamea is found growing in America and Canada and was traditionally used by the American Indians for medicinal and religious purposes and was reputed to be the biblical 'Balm of Gilead'. The sturdiness and height of this Fir gives it grounding qualities while the strong green energy brings great healing to the heart. On a physical level, Fir essential oil has a therapeutic action on the lungs and respiratory system, relieving congestion in the lungs. The strength of the energy has a tonic effect on our whole system, bringing the invigorating effect of oxygen from the air, and light energy from the ether. Like other oils with a sympathetic resonance with green, Fir has a freeing action on the mind and emotions giving us space to just be and think, without making decisions or taking action. It brings the emotions back into balance in situations where one feels trapped and repressed by other people.

Therapeutic uses	Aromatherapy	Colour therapy
Physical	benefits the respiratory and immune system	green to chest and throat
	use for acute asthma	green to chest and throat
	invigorating to the muscles, and good for aches and pains, arthritis, rheumatism	green inhalation, compresses
Emotional	heals the heart in times of shock, grief	green to heart chakra
	freeing action when feeling trapped	green to heart chakra
	gives you emotional space	green colour breathing
Mental	relieves a tired mind	green colour breathing
	allows time to think and consider	green inhalation, green to brow chakra

| *Spiritual* | grounding while allowing love to flow | green to whole body |
| | cleansing to the aura, bringing balance | green to whole body |

Precautions: non-toxic, non-irritant (but use in small doses), non-sensitising

Affirmations: With the deep green energy of Fir, I can open myself to universal love and have the freedom to choose my next course of action.

FRANKINCENSE
BOSWELLIA CARTERI/THURIFERA
Healing colours/s: violet and gold
Colour aroma treatment/s: colour compresses, foot baths using gold-coloured towels, colour inhaler, perfumes, solarised creams, beauty lotions
Chakra affinity: crown
Life qualities: purification, dignity, cleansed, restoration, balance, protection

Colour signature: Frankincense has many ancient associations, dating back to before Biblical times. The oil is made by making incisions in the bark of the tree which exudes a resin in yellow drops or tears. The essential oil is a product of steam distillation of the tears. It has been traditionally used as a fumigant and to ward off evil spirits and this is because the violet vibrations emitted by Frankincense are of a high frequency which creates a protective force field around one. The violet in Frankincense soothes and purifies at all levels and deepens and slows the breath. It has a cleansing effect on the lungs by removing mucus and the red in the violet ray helps the action of the genito-urinary tract. Frankincense is often mixed with cinnamon, another yellow oil, and applied to aching limbs. Violet has a regenerative and healing action which encourages the growth of new cells and the formation of scar tissue and it has been reputed for keeping the skin smooth, supple and hydrated. The harmonising yellow ray also purges the lymphatic system, and removing toxins from the body.

Therapeutic uses	Aromatherapy	Colour therapy
Physical	uterine haemorrhages, heavy periods	violet light therapy to reflexes of feet.
	drains lymphatics	violet to lymphatic areas
	aching limbs, healing wounds, burns,	violet and yellow to affected area
	removes mucus from the lungs	violet to the chest
Emotional	slows down breathing and brings a feeling of calmness	violet light therapy to base chakra
	complete acceptance and understanding	violet to the heart chakra
Mental	elevating and soothing effect on the mind	violet on the crown chakra
	helps connection to higher mind through meditation and opening the crown chakra	violet to crown chakra
Spiritual	releases anxiety and obsessions linked to the past. A spiritual teacher.	violet over the crown chakra

Precautions: None known.

Affirmations: The violet ray lets me release all harmful vibrations from the past.
Frankincense brings violet to my system so I can relax and calm my mind.

GARLIC

ALLIUM SATIVUM

Healing colours/s: pink and white
Colour aroma treatment/s: capsules, colour aromatic cooking, colour
visualisation and meditation
Chakra affinity: heart and crown
Life qualities: strength, courage, forgiveness, good health and longevity

Colour signature: Garlic is familiar plant whose white bulbs are used widely
in cooking and which are reputed to bestow strength and longevity. A garlic
plant can grow up to three feet and has white/pink flowers and long flat
leaves. The oil made from garlic is colourless with a strong smell of garlic,
and for this reason most people prefer to take it internally in capsule form.
Being a bulb, Garlic contains red, magnetic earth energy, which is mixed
with white light in the flowers to give a deep pink colour signature. The
pink ray stimulates the reproductive system while simultaneously
opening the heart chakra so that love can flow. The soft green leaves
compliment the qualities of the pink ray. Its protective qualities also come
from its pink and white colour signature. White light is a very fast
vibration which has the power to create a shield of protection by
energising the forcefield in the aura. This is the underlying reason why
garlic has a long history of use against psychic and physical attack.

Therapeutic uses	Aromatherapy	Colour therapy
Physical	reduces blood pressure and thins blood, helps rheumatic pains	pink to soles of feet
	detoxifies the body by toning the lymphatic system,	pink to whole body
	helps dissolve skin congestion and allergies, disinfectant	pink to whole body
	natural anti-biotic	pink to whole body, white colour breathing
	stimulates the flow of bile to the gall-bladder	pink to gall-bladder

Emotional	releases bitter resentment by purging the gall-bladder	pink to heart chakra, colour breathing
	helps one forgive and find compassion for others	pink to heart chakra
Mental	warming and stimulating to the mind	pink to whole body
	good for apathy and disinterest in life	pink to brown chakra
Spiritual	cleanses Ch'i in the kidneys, purifies the dross of accumulated Karma	pink to kidneys
	psychic protection	white visualisation

Precautions: Do not use on fiery temperaments, or if suffering from eczema or heated conditions. Nursing mothers should avoid.

Affirmations: With the love and protection of Garlic I can lead a long healthy life.

GERANIUM
Pelargonium graveolens/odorantissimum
Healing colours/s: green and pink
Colour aroma treatment/s: colour baths, colour massage, spray mists, skin preparations, colour aroma lamps and room diffusers
Chakra affinity: heart
Life qualities: healing, harmonious, comforting, tranquil, sensitive, open

Colour signature: Geranium is an aromatic shrub with serrated leaves and small pink flowers which have an apple-like aroma. The strong green vibration in Geranium makes it a wonderfully healing oil which promotes inner balance necessary for speedy recuperation after an illness or operation. It has a regulatory effect on our system, normalising metabolism, harmonising the mind and emotions, which makes it wonderful for the treatment of stress. The cleansing effect of green energy clears out the digestive system and dispels mucus from the lungs, and also disposes of waste products especially where there is water retention. The gentle action of the pink ray is nurturing and comforting to the heart, signalling a new beginning for love. The harmonious vibrations in Geranium, stimulates the flow of blood which has a beneficial effect on the complexion and skin in general.

Therapeutic uses	Aromatherapy	Colour therapy
Physical	cooling and soothing to a sore throat, tonsillitis	green over throat
	promotes healing to bruises, broken capillaries, cuts, ulcers, wounds	green over the affected area
	cleansing and toning to mature skin, oily skin balances oily and dry skins	green to lungs and liver
	cellulite, poor circulation	green over legs, hips, stomach
Emotional	comforts and heals the heart, PMS and menopausal problems	green light on heart chakra
	relieves nervous tension	as above
	soothes and calms and brings feelings of peace and tranquillity	green light irradiation of whole body
Mental	lightens the mood, good for neuralgia, stress, anxiety and depression	green over crown and through feet
	connects heart to higher mind	green over heart and crown

| *Spiritual* | helps release creative blocks by opening the heart to the flow of universal love, protection against negative forces | green over crown |

Precautions: non-toxic, non-irritant, non-sensitising, caution when used on sensitive skins. Avoid in pregnancy.

Affirmations: With the green ray, Geranium balances and harmonises my whole system. Geranium protects me from harmful vibrations so that I am restful and happy.

GINGER

ZINGIBER OFFICINALE

Healing colours/s: orange and golden yellow
Colour aroma treatment/s: colour massage, colour-aroma lamp, colour compresses, colour aroma breathing, colour aromatic drinks
Chakra affinity: sacral, throat
Life qualities: spiritual, enlightened, protective, knowledgeable, wise

Colour signature: The orange colour signature of this herb is taken from the earthy quality of its rhizome root, which produces a mustard yellow colour powder when dried and powdered. Ginger, like its colour frequency is best known as a digestive aid, and for its ability to release coldness and mucus from the system. Ginger has also been used since ancient times as an aphrodisiac and remedy for impotence. On an emotional level the orange energy makes it stimulating, yet grounding and aids release of tears. It gives us self-confidence allowing us to be more assertive in expressing our real thoughts and feelings. The yellow energy also found in Ginger focuses the mind so we can think clearly helping us with decision-making. The golden-yellow of wisdom is attracted through inner communication with the higher mind.

Therapeutic uses	Aromatherapy	Colour therapy
Physical	colic, cramp, flatulence, indigestion, loss of appetite, nausea	yellow over liver
	chills, colds, flu, fever	orange over sacral chakra
	congestion in the lungs coughs, sinusitis, sore throat	orange over chest
	poor circulation, fatigue, aches and pains, helps clear bruises	orange over base, blue over bruises
Emotional	stimulating and uplifting	orange over sacral area
	cheering when emotionally worn out	
	renews romantic interest	orange to sacral centre
	teaches acceptance where there has been a constant struggle to fight	violet to heart and crown chakras
Mental	sharpens the mind and aids memory	yellow over solar-plexus
Spiritual	energises the aura lifting vibrations and bringing transformation, enlightenment and inspiration	violet to crown, meditation, breathing

Precautions: non-toxic, may irritate sensitive skins, slightly photo-toxic

Affirmations: The orange ray in Ginger removes unwanted liquids from my system. With the orange ray, I release all negative vibrations and live joyously.

GRAPEFRUIT

Citrus paradisi
Healing colours/s: yellow and violet
Colour aroma treatment/s: colour massage, colour aroma bath, colour
breathing, colour aroma skin preparations, solarised water
Chakra affinity: solar-plexus and crown
Life qualities: inspired, attuned, radiating, cheerful, liberated

Colour signature: Grapefruit is a clear or water-white oil which is made by cold expression from the fresh peel. The tree from which it comes is large with glossy leaves and large yellow fruit. The oil's affinity with yellow makes it resonant with the digestive and nervous system. Yellow light has the ability to cleanse and purify by its releasing action, making Grapefruit excellent for helping lymphatic drainage and the elimination of toxins from the body, particularly through the skin. Its effect on the nervous system is strengthening, which in turn stimulates the mental processes. Its tonic affect on the nervous system is useful for alleviating stress and nervous exhaustion. The clear yellow vibration in Grapefruit is the colour of the sun, which helps lift depression and develop a more positive outlook. The yellow also attracts its complementary energy, Violet, which purifies the emotions and mind bringing a feeling of release from restrictions leading to spiritual purity.

Therapeutic uses	Aromatherapy	Colour therapy
Physical	acne, oily skin, hair growth, toning to skin and tissues stiffness, muscle fatigue, cellulite, obesity, water retention	yellow light irradiation to whole body yellow light to affected area
	colds, flu, chills headaches	yellow light to feet yellow light to solar-plexus

Emotional	eases grief caused by emotional or mental violence	violet to crown chakra
	brings comfort during pregnancy, relieves PMT	yellow irradiation to whole body
	helps one cope with feelings of resentment and envy	
	promotes self-confidence and dissipates fears	yellow light to solar-plexus
Mental	uplifting for severe depression, brings alertness, feeling connected, inspired	yellow light to solar-plexus
	opens up new possibilities and new ideas	yellow light to solar-plexus
Spiritual	euphoric and hypnotic qualities aid relaxation of the conscious mind.	colour breathing, colour aroma lamp while relaxing

Precautions: None known.

Affirmations: The yellow grapefruit protects me against all infection. The yellow ray opens up my mind so I can see new possibilities.

HYSSOP
HYSSOPUS OFFICINALIS
Healing colours/s: blue and violet
Colour aroma treatment/s: spray mists, colour compresses, colour aromatic cooking, colour aroma lamps, room diffusers, perfumes, colour breathing
Chakra affinity: throat, brow, crown
Life qualities: purification, invigoration, healing

161

Colour signature: Hyssop is an elegant almost evergreen shrub with a woody stem, and slender lance-shaped leaves. It has blue-purple flowers, which are particularly attractive to bees and give the oil its blue colour signature. The astringent and purifying qualities of both the blue and violet rays make Hyssop especially healing to the skin helping form scars, clearing bruising, dermatitis and eczema. The power of Hyssop to promote rapid healing has also seen its use in the treatment of cancerous growths. Hyssop also has the pain-relieving qualities of deep blue, and it is useful for curing grief by releasing emotional pain which is held in the spleen. The sedating action on the nervous system and mind makes Hyssop beneficial for the treatment of all anxieties and nervous complaints especially hysteria and emotional trauma. By linking us to our intuition, the deep blue ray helps inner communication so we can really come to know ourselves.

Therapeutic uses	Aromatherapy	Colour therapy
Physical	raises low blood pressure	violet to soles of feet or whole body
	use externally on wound, bruises, cuts and for toothache, earache	colour aroma compresses
	soothing and reducing inflammation	colour aroma compresses
Emotional	releasing emotional pain by inner cleansing	violet to heart chakra
	treating grief through transformation	violet to the crown chakra
Mental	balances the psyche	violet to the brow chakra
	sedative to the mind making it easier to connect with one's intuition and creativity	violet to the crown chakra

| *Spiritual* | spiritual cleansing and healing | violet to whole aura, perfume |
| | purification and protection of the environment | violet spray mist, candle, colour aroma lamp, visualisation |

Precautions: Avoid during pregnancy, of if you suffer from epilepsy or high blood pressure.

Affirmations: With the violet ray of Hyssop I am purified and cleansed of all negative vibrations within my system.

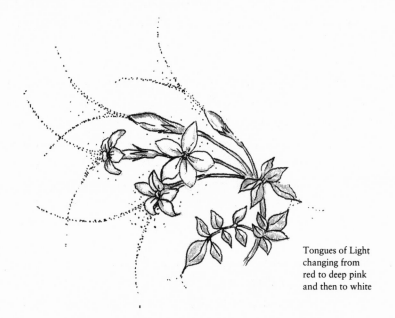

Tongues of Light changing from red to deep pink and then to white

JASMINE

JASMINUM GRANDIFLORUM

Healing colours/s: white, red, deep pink
Colour aroma treatment/s: colour bath, room diffuser, colour massage, scented candles, garlands, perfumes
Chakra affinity: base and sacral
Life qualities: self-awareness, confidence, sensuality, openness, connection, inspiration

Colour signature: Jasmine is an evergreen shrub or climber which is native to China and has a sweet pervasive scent and small white star-shaped flowers. Its dark orange brown oil is intensely warm and richly scented and has been used traditionally as an aphrodisiac, for hard contracted limbs, reproductive and nervous problems. The colour orange is a wonderful anti-depressant which has the capacity to instil confidence and optimism. The base and sacral area link strongly with the sexual organs, and Jasmine connects more to female problems in the genito-urinary system. On an emotional and spiritual level, Jasmine has the reputation of bringing happiness and peace. Its red ray promotes self-confidence and assertiveness because we know who we are and are happy with ourselves. The white flowers lift the red vibrations to a deep rose pink which opens our hearts so we become more sensitive and compassionate by linking to the force of universal love. This helps us develop our creativity and self-expression bringing more joy into our lives. The star shape of the white flowers floods the aura with white light, transmuting the energy of the base chakra to a higher level.

Therapeutic uses	Aromatherapy	Colour therapy
Physical	coughs with tightness in the chest, laryngitis	pink over pelvis, or chest
	good for a dry skin, by warming and relaxing tension	pink over whole body
	muscular spasms, frigidity, labour pains, uterine disorders	pink over lower back and pelvis
Emotional	releases emotions and helps us move on from past pain.	pink over heart
	teaches you tactile enjoyment	pink over sacral centre
	Calms nerves, gives confidence, warms emotions	pink over solar-plexus
Mental	Anti-depressant, fights apathy, lack of interest in life, listlessness	red over the base chakra

| *Spiritual* | Grounding, teaching you joyous connection with your body | red over the base chakra or soles of the feet |

Precautions: non-toxic, non-irritant, usually non-sensitising. Avoid in pregnancy.

Affirmations: With the orange ray I am confident and happily living in the present.
With the red ray, I express my sexuality with love and joy.

JUNIPER
JUNIPERUS COMMUNIS
Healing colours/s: violet
Colour aroma treatment/s: colour aroma diffuser, spray mists, colour poultices and compresses, colour breathing, perfumes, colour soaps and lotions
Chakra affinity: crown and base
Life qualities: vision, sacredness, humility, conviction, service, cleansing

Colour signature: Juniper is a large evergreen shrub with long dark needles. It is native to the south of France and is found throughout Europe and North Africa. Juniper takes its colour signature from its blue-violet berries which are about the same size as hazelnuts and often used in cooking. Its violet colour signature gives it purifying and cleansing properties as well as stimulating properties increasing blood supply to the cells and tissues. It therefore makes a good oil for the treatment of skin diseases such as eczema and scalp problems including hair loss. Its antiseptic qualities are also useful for the treatment of wounds, cuts and sores and for cleansing the environment of harmful vibrations. As violet light contains both red and blue energy, Juniper gives us emotional support and strength while we pursue our aims with sincerity and humility. The sacred nature of Juniper allows us to see the beauty and truth in all things both external and internal bringing us spiritual knowledge and understanding.

Therapeutic uses	Aromatherapy	Colour therapy
Physical	purifies and has antiseptic properties. Use for skin care, skin toner, wounds, acne, eczema, hair loss	violet over affected area
	anti-viral for colds, flu, infections, detoxifies and purges the system, use for cellulitis, gout, obesity, rheumatism	violet over chest violet through the crown and feet
	cystitis, haemorrhoids	violet on the pelvis
Emotional	helps us accept emotional violence, dissolves guilt and fears of facing death, feelings of worthlessness	violet through the crown and solar-plexus
Mental	purifies the mind and helps with addictions, obsessions, confusion, restlessness	violet through the crown
Spiritual	helps one withdraw and become an observer of life, bringing peace and wisdom	violet through the crown

Precautions: non-toxic, non-irritant, check skin allergic reactions before use.

Affirmations: With the Violet ray, my hair is healthy, soft and luxuriant. The violet ray flowing through Juniper supports my mind and spirit.

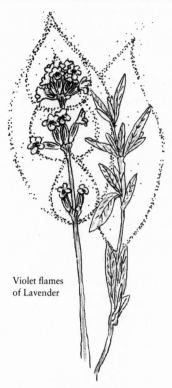

Violet flames
of Lavender

LAVENDER

LAVENDULA OFFICINALIS
Healing colours/s: violet
Colour aroma treatment/s: colour aroma massage, colour bath, spray
mist, lotions and skin care preparations, solar-charged water, colour
compresses, colour aroma lamps, colour breathing, perfume, colour
inhalation, candles, meditation
Chakra affinity: crown and base
Life qualities: rejuvenation, protection, reconcilation, balance

Colour signature: This woody evergreen shrub is probably the most widely
used healing plant throughout history. It was known by the Romans for
its skin healing properties and for cleansing of infectious diseases, plague,
convulsions, epilepsy, fainting and all pains in the head. Its penetrating high
violet vibration comes from the beautiful violet-blue flowers which point
upwards, as if lifting energy to the sky. The stems of the plant are covered
with star-shaped hairs and narrow grey-green leaves, and the essential oil
has a colourless appearance instilling it with white light. Lavender has a

sedating effect on the heart thus lowering blood pressure. Its calming and uplifting vibrations bring relief from pain and fears of the mind. The violet vibration allows us to stand back from life so that we disassociate ourselves from our emotions. In this way we become aware of a higher consciousness and our spiritual nature.

Therapeutic uses	Aromatherapy	Colour therapy
Physical	lowers blood pressure, heart sedative	violet on soles of feet
	promotes new cell growth, heals burns, scars	violet over affected area
	acne, eczema, psoriasis, boils, swellings	violet on affected area
	eases muscular spasm by stimulating venous blood flow, use for rheumatic pain, varicose veins	violet through soles of feet, legs, hands
	stimulates endocrine system, good for nausea, vomiting, flatulence, aids digestion of fats	violet over spleen or spleen and liver foot reflex
	respiratory problems,	violet over chest
	scanty and painful periods	violet to lower abdomen
Emotional	emotionally comforting, calms anger, soothes anxieties, apprehension, breakdown, fear of change, moodiness, facing death, hysteria, panic attacks	violet to crown and heart
Mental	resolves conflicts in the mind. Use for delirium, irritability, mental exhaustion, dementia, manic-depression, phobias, insomnia	violet over crown and soles of the feet

Spiritual	spiritual growth by producing a meditative state	violet to brown and crown
	stabilises physical, etheric and astral bodies, psychic protection	violet on crown and feet or whole body light irradiation

Precautions: Avoid during early pregnancy, and if you have low blood pressure.

Affirmations: The violet ray fills my whole body with light and peace.

LEMON
Citrus limonum
Healing colours/s: yellow and green
Colour aroma treatment/s: colour baths, colour massage, colour aroma room spray, aroma colour breathing, solar charged water, coloured floral water
Chakra affinity: solar-plexus
Life qualities: lively, extroverted, direct, humorous, versatile, conscious

Colour signature: The small thorny evergreen Lemon tree has shiny oval leaves and pink and white flowers. The fruits are green turning yellow when ripe. The essential oil is a better quality when made from the unripe fruits so the colour vibrations will vary accordingly. (Check with a pendulum). The yellow colour signature of lemon links it with the endocrine system, so lemon essential oil, which contains a high dosage of Vitamin C, is a tonic for the whole glandular system. It has long been regarded as a rejuvenator and 'cure all' for infectious diseases. Yellow is the colour which has a cleansing and purifying action on the digestive system, so this oil is a useful tonic for the liver and kidneys and for cleansing the pancreas. Its releasing action liquefies the blood, thus bringing down high blood pressure and aiding the flow in varicose veins. Lemon is an essential oil which builds up the strength by stimulating the production of white blood corpuscles. The mind and central nervous system has a sympathetic vibration to yellow, so Lemon is useful for treatment of neuralgia, headaches, and migraine due to nervous tension. Lemon helps focus the mind and is a good oil for meditation. It also works on the solar-plexus to build up personal power and confidence helping us develop a more positive outlook.

Therapeutic uses	Aromatherapy	Colour therapy
Physical	aids circulation, heart tonic, restores vitality	yellow to soles of the feet
	soothes sore throats, coughs, flu when accompanied with a high temperature	yellow to abdomen and chest
	counteracts acidity in stomach, stimulates pancreas, cellulite	yellow to liver area
Emotional	calms and refreshes when you are hot and bothered, irritable counteracts feelings of resentment and bitterness helps you develop a more positive outlook	yellow light or scarf over the solar-plexus yellow to solar-plexus and gall-bladder
Mental	focuses the mind, aids clear thinking, concentration, improves performance and decision-making	yellow light to solar-plexus
Spiritual	Useful for meditation, creativity and joy, love of life	aroma colour lamp or candle, colour breathing

Precautions: non-toxic, photo-toxic when skin exposed directly to sunlight, use with caution on sensitive skin.

Affirmations: With the yellow ray in Lemon I am cool and clear headed.

LEMONGRASS

Cymbopogon citratus

Healing colours/s: yellow
Colour aroma treatment/s: colour breathing, perfume spray mist, colour aroma lamp diffuser, colour massage (use with caution), solarised food and drink, insecticide, aroma candle
Chakra affinity: solar- plexus
Life qualities: flexibility, wisdom, determination, clarity of thought, perception, discrimination

Colour signature: Cultivated from a wild grass, Lemongrass takes its colour signature from the long yellow stem and leaves. Its oil varies between a yellow and amber colour with a fresh grassy citrus aroma. Lemongrass has a strong affinity with yellow and therefore is a tonic and stimulant to the nervous system. Its toning and cleansing properties make it good for the treatment of relaxed muscles and poor circulation. It has a beneficial action on the digestive system and like other yellow oils is a good treatment for fevers and infectious diseases. The real benefit of Lemongrass lies in its sedative action on the nerves, and the treatment of stress, related to nervous tension and exhaustion. Its mentally stimulating properties make it similar to Lemon in its ability to help clear and focus the mind while allowing one to remain flexible. This enables us to make wise judgements, not from the ego but by accessing the universal mind.

Therapeutic uses	Aromatherapy	Colour therapy
Physical	muscular aches and pains, poor circulation, promotes muscle tone	yellow light to affected area, legs and feet.
	acne, open pores, oily skin, athlete's foot, scabies	yellow light to stomach and upper abdomen
	indigestion, gastro-enteritis	yellow light to stomach
	infections with fever	yellow light to feet

Emotional	tonic to the nerves, use for stress, helps establish personal power	yellow scarf or light to solar-plexus
Mental	mental stimulant, focus, concentration and clarity of vision	yellow light to solar-plexus and feet
Spiritual	inspiration and brings wisdom into one's affairs	gold to crown chakra
	promotes wise judgement	candle light with aroma bath

Precautions: non-toxic, use with care on sensitive skin, use low dosage. Maximum of 1%.

Affirmations: With the yellow ray of Lemongrass my muscles are strengthening and toning. The yellow ray restores my personal power so that I can be more assertive.

LIME

Citrus medica/aurantifolia
Healing colours/s: green
Colour aroma treatment/s: colour baths, spray mists, colour compresses, colour aromatic cooking, colour aroma lamps, room diffusers, perfumes, colour breathing,
Chakra affinity: heart
Life qualities: focusing, clarity, aware, calm, balanced, compassionate

Colour signature: This small evergreen tree has smooth ovate leaves and small white flowers. The essence is made from the peel of the unripe fruit which has a pale green colouring and is bitter to the taste. The oil is also usually a pale yellow-green in colour with a sharp citrus scent. Lime has the therapeutic properties of the green ray, cleansing and purifying at all levels and its healing properties make it useful to aid speedy recuperation.

It is astringent to the skin and stimulates circulation by helping eliminate toxins and excess water from the body. The green colour signature helps soothe and balance the emotions and psyche by its cleansing and restorative action. It brings alertness to the mind and renews interest in life.

Therapeutic uses	Aromatherapy	Colour therapy
Physical	reduces fevers, wards off infections	green to whole body
	stimulates circulation	yellow to soles of feet
	good for all respiratory problems, asthma, catarrh, throat infections	green to chest and throat
	immune tonic, gives energy after illness	green to whole body
	cleansing and toning to an oily skin, use for spots, warts, mouth ulcers	green to liver, gall-bladder, lungs
Emotional	balances the emotions and promotes self-love	green to heart chakra
	brings calmness and compassion	green to heart chakra
Mental	uplifting to the tired mind	yellow to solar-plexus chakra
	helps redress apathy, anxiety and depression	yellow to crown chakra
	promotes alertness and stimulates mind in cases of mental debility (Dementia)	yellow and green to feet
Spiritual	balances addictions by purging the aura of negative and harmful vibrations	green to whole body
	harmonises the energy in all the chakras	green to solar-plexus

Precautions: May irritate a sensitive skin.

Affirmations: With the uplifting green ray in Lime, I am aware, alert and focused.

LINDEN BLOSSOM
TILIA EUROPAEA
Healing colours/s: green
Colour aroma treatment/s: colour spray mists, colour aroma lamps, colour inhalant, colour sleepy-time pillow, colour massage
Chakra affinity: heart
Life qualities: gentleness, serenity, security, patience, stability

Colour signature: This large tree has dull grey bark with dark green serrated and heart-shaped leaves which are light green below. Its flowers are yellow white and pendulous with a powerful scent. Linden takes its colour signature from its heart-shaped green leaves, as it links strongly with the heart chakra which it opens, bringing back self-esteem and release from guilt or possessiveness. The oil is widely used for the treatment of arteriosclerotic hypertension and it helps clear cholesterol and chronic circulatory diseases. Green has a cleansing and diuretic action and Linden clears out the kidneys, moving excess urea from the system. It is also useful for the treatment of rheumatism and gout. This relaxing oil promotes sleep and has a calming effect on the emotions, especially in cases of anger, hysteria and mood swings. The loving quality of the green and pink ray make Linden a good oil for those people who are grieving, suffering loss or rejection as it promotes self-love and self-esteem.

Therapeutic uses	Aromatherapy	Colour therapy
Physical	chronic catarrh, flu, pleurisy, bronchitis, fevers through sweating	green over chest
	detoxifies kidneys, liver	green over kidneys, liver
	stomach, indigestion, diarrhoea	
	rheumatism, gout	green to soles of feet
Emotional	balances emotions, calms anger, helps cope with loss, rejection, grief, releases emotional blocks	green to heart chakra
	emotional burn-out, hysteria, phobias and mood swings	as above
Mental	relaxing to the mind, helps sleep, migraine	green to base and crown
Spiritual	provides stability and balance allowing inner growth	green to heart chakra
	gives you space to be calm and heal	green to heart chakra

Precautions: non-toxic, may irritate sensitive skins

Affirmations: Linden brings me freedom to breathe deeply and trust in the process of life. Green energy fills my body brings harmony and balance to every part of me.

MANDARIN

CITRUS MADURENSIS/RETICULATA

Healing colours/s: orange and blue
Colour aroma treatment/s: colour massage, colour aroma bath, colour aroma lamp, spray mists, perfumes
Chakra affinity: sacral
Life qualities: inspired, refreshed, sympathetic, creative expression, intuitive

Colour signature: The Mandarin is a small evergreen tree with bright glossy leaves and fragrant flowers. Its fruit is orange coloured and fleshy. The oil is a yellow-orange colour with a blue-violet hint and has a very citrus-sweet aroma. The strong orange colour signature of the oil makes it good for treatment of congestion in the skin, and its releasing quality helps elasticity which is good for promoting the formation of scar tissue, reducing stretch marks and toning an oily skin. Mandarin is a good digestive and is invaluable for boosting the digestive system of the elderly. Like all orange oils, Mandarin helps move excess fluid from the body. The orange ray reflected by the oil helps develop self-awareness and a good self-image and the positive vibrations attract joy and happiness. The complementary colours of blue and orange open the sacral and throat chakras which work together encouraging release of deep emotions by giving them creative and verbal expression.

Level of healing	Aromatherapy	Colour therapy
Physical	fluid retention and obesity	orange light over the
	diarrhoea due to nervous tension	pituitary reflex on the foot
	intestinal and digestive problems	orange light over the stomach and pelvis
	stimulates appetite when loss of hunger due to depression	orange light to abdomen

Emotional	helps treat anxiety and the feeling of emptiness. Helps counteract shyness	orange followed by blue light over the solar-plexus
	helps release the past, comforts the inner child nurturing of inner emotional desires	orange to sacral and blue to throat chakra
Mental	insomnia, nervous tension, restlessness	blue light over the back of the head
Spiritual	lifts spirits and connects to intuition,	blue to throat and brow, orange to sacral
	strengthens through purifying the aura, inner communication	orange light through the soles of the feet

Precautions: Non-toxic, non-irritant, non-sensitising, sometimes phototoxic.

Affirmations: Mandarin brings warmth and joy into my life. With the orange ray my skin is healing so that no scar remains.

MARIGOLD
CALENDULA OFFICINALIS
Healing colours/s: yellow and green
Colour aroma treatment/s: colour baths, colour massage, spray mists, colour compresses, colour aromatic cooking, colour aroma lamps, room diffusers, perfumes, colour breathing, lotions and skin creams, meditation
Chakra affinity: solar-plexus, heart
Life qualities: radiant, loving, wise, bright, communicative, quick-witted

Colour signature: Marigold is an annual herb that has pale green leaves and bright orange daisy-like flowers. The absolute is extracted from the flowers and produces a greeny-brown liquid with a sharp herbaceous aroma. The radial shape of the flowers together with their strong colouring

177

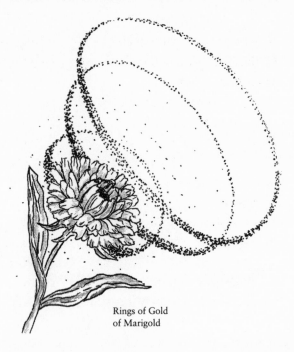

Rings of Gold
of Marigold

makes Marigold a joyous and uplifting oil. Yellow and green have cleansing properties, and Marigold is an ancient remedy for healing wounds and sores and for the treatment of many skin problems when used as external compresses. The underlying green energy gives the oil its anti-septic, astringent and anti-inflammatory qualities which makes its useful to combat fevers and also burns and rashes. Marigold has also been used to treat inflamed lymph nodes and duodenal ulcers. The golden ray in this oil opens up our soul to spiritual wisdom and the abundance of the universe.

Level of healing	Aromatherapy	Colour therapy
Physical	use for skin care, cuts, wounds, burns and inflammations	yellow/green externally as compresses
	assists menstruation and other menstrual problems	yellow to pelvis
	useful for varicose veins	yellow to affected area

Emotional	opens the heart promoting communication through a strong sense of self	yellow to heart chakra and solar-plexus
	helps let go of the past and rejoice in the present	yellow to sacral chakra
	helps connect with our inner sun promoting self-confidence and esteem	yellow to solar-plexus and hara (navel)
Mental	uplifting, bringing the golden-ray of wisdom	yellow to crown chakra, colour breathing
	calming but also a tonic to the mind	yellow to solar-plexus
Spiritual	brightness attracts prosperity and abundance	green to crown
	allows the radiance of the soul to shine through	gold to heart centre, visualisation

Precautions: Avoid during pregnancy.

Affirmations: With the radiance of Marigold, I feel the power of my own inner sun.

MARJORAM

ORIGANUM MARJORANA

Healing colours/s: blue and orange
Colour aroma treatment/s: colour massage, colour baths, solar-charged lotions and creams, colour poultices and compresses, colour breathing
Chakra affinity: throat and sacral
Life qualities: restful, restored, confident, restraint, sincere, creative, courageous

Colour signature: The bushy aromatic Sweet Marjoram is a tender plant with dark green leaves and small greyish white flowers. The oil is a pale yellow or amber colour which has an affinity with both blue and orange vibrations. The blue gives it its soothing quality, while the orange brings it warming and fortifying effects. It comforts cold diseases in the stomach, head, and chest, releasing obstructions in the liver and spleen. The orange signature works on the blood, clearing bruising by easing blood flow. It also dilates the arteries and capillaries, thus bringing a feeling of well-being and warmth throughout the system. The blue ray prevents tissue degeneration, arrests bleeding in wounds and gives it pain healing qualities. Its soothing vibrations help soothe away troubles and comfort those suffering from recent grief or bereavement. Marjoram was thought to bring peace to departed spirits, and it can bring acceptance and understanding to those who face death.

Level of healing	Aromatherapy	Colour therapy
Physical	painful muscles, backache, rheumatic pain, swollen joints, bruises	blue over affected area
	digestive problems	blue over abdomen
	soothes digestion, cramps, constipation, flatulence	blue of stomach and bowel
	chest infections, colds	blue and orange over chest
Emotional	clears deep emotional traumas, comforts grieving, loneliness	blue and orange over throat and sacral chakra
	helps us confront issues so we can heal	orange to sacral and solar-plexus
Mental	delirium, relieves anxieties, stress, hyperactive people, addiction	blue over crown or through feet

| *Spiritual* | brings you in touch with your intuition | blue over throat |
| | bringer of good fortune, longevity and peace to departed spirits | blue to whole aura |

Precautions: non-toxic, non-sensitising, non-irritant, can cause drowsiness, avoid during pregnancy.

Affirmations: Marjoram contains the blue ray which restores calm and enables me to relax fully. The blue vibration dispels my fears so I can enjoy peaceful sleep.

MELISSA (Lemon Balm)
MELISSA OFFICINALIS
Healing colours/s: pink and green
Colour aroma treatment/s: colour fragrance burner, colour breathing, solarised tea or water, sleepy colour pillow. (green and pink pillow filled with herbs placed under your pillow at night)
Chakra affinity: heart
Life qualities: constancy, affection, composure, tranquillity, nurture, comfort

Colour signature: Melissa, also known as Lemon Balm, is a sweet-scented bushy herb with bright green serrated leaves and tiny white and pink flowers. The oil is a pale yellow colour with a lemon scent. Melissa has an affinity with the heart chakra as it contains the calming effect of green energy. It balances high blood pressure by relaxing the heart muscles. The pink ray in Melissa harmonises with the female reproductive system and the green and pink work together to help with painful menstruation, a tonic effect on the uterus which is beneficial to conception difficulties. Lemon Balm also reflects the green-yellow wave length which harmonises the solar-plexus chakra. The yellow element of Lemon balm has a beneficial effect on the digestive system and central nervous system relieving stress due to anxiety and hypertension. Melissa works through the feminine aspect with the pink ray helping us develop self-love, so that we can learn to nurture ourselves as well as others. Once we love ourselves and not rely on others to love us first, we are filled with a deep sense of peace and tranquillity.

Level of healing	Aromatherapy	Colour therapy
Physical	treatment of asthma, bronchitis, coughs	green light over the heart
	indigestion, colic, nausea, dysentery, flatulence	green over the liver
	menstrual pain, tonic to the uterus, helps conception	pink over the pelvis and heart
	skin care, insect bites, allergies, eczema	green to affected area
Emotional	calming yet uplifting effect on the emotions, helps in grieving, soothes panic, shock and for people who are hypersensitive	pink followed by green over the heart
Mental	helps promote a positive outlook, lifts depression by releasing mental blocks and nervous tension	pink light over solar-plexus
Spiritual	Teaches you the lesson that everything comes in its own time	green over the heart chakra

Precautions: non-toxic, may irritate a sensitive skin, avoid during pregnancy.

Affirmations: The pink ray of Melissa allows me to release my pain and allows love into my life. With the green ray I feel myself relaxing and I take life as it comes.

MYRRH

COMMIPHORA MYRRHA

Healing colours/s: red / deep pink (red with white)
Colour aroma treatment/s: colour baths, colour massage, spray mists, colour compresses, colour aromatic cooking, colour aroma lamps, aromatic candles, room diffusers, perfumes, colour breathing, incense
Chakra affinity: base and crown
Life qualities: commitment, will, stability, patience, resolution, selfless love

Colour signature: Myrrh is a small tree with knotted branches and aromatic leaves and white flowers. The oil is resinous and a deep reddish brown, giving Myrrh a strong red colour signature which has a strong affinity with the base chakra. The red ray in Myrrh contains warming and stimulating properties which have a releasing effect on all parts of our system. On a physical level, red warms the genito-urinary system and is a tonic to the stomach. Its strengthening action stimulates the spleen to produce white blood corpuscles building up the immune system. It was a favourite oil in ancient times for use in embalming because of its ability to preserve the skin. Its action on the skin is one of relaxing the muscles and giving the skin elasticity, thus making it a useful component of skin creams and moisturisers. The white energy pervading the oil gives Myrrh the ability to balance the subtle bodies and polarise the energy in the base and crown chakras. The red ray strengthens spirituality and revitalises life force energy within us.

Level of healing	Aromatherapy	Colour therapy
Physical	good for chronic respiratory problems	pink to the chest
	stimulates the appetite and digestion	red to the abdomen
	strengthens physical weakness allowing one to become physically active	red to the soles of the feet
	good for a mature skin and wrinkles	pink to the affected area
	also treatment of wounds and fungal infections	

Emotional	promotes inner security and stability	red to the base chakra
	helps those with an inferiority complex or with a need to control others	red to the base chakra
Mental	strengthens the mind giving one purpose, perseverance and motivation	red to the solar-plexus
Spiritual	strengthens spirituality by opening the base chakra, allowing life force energy to flow into the kidneys	red to the base chakra
	polarises the base and crown chakras	pink to whole body, or feet and crown

Precautions: Avoid during pregnancy. Do not use red light above the chest or on anyone suffering from heart problems or high blood pressure.

Affirmations: With the red ray of Myrrh I walk purposefully down my path in life.

MYRTLE
MYRTUS COMMUNIS
Healing colours/s: Blue, green (turquoise), indigo
Colour aroma treatment/s: colour baths, colour massage, spray mists, colour compresses, colour aromatic cooking, colour aroma lamps, room diffusers, perfumes, colour breathing, colour reflexology, skin lotions and tonics.
Chakra affinity: heart, throat and thymus
Life qualities: peace, love, insight, understanding, refinement, perception

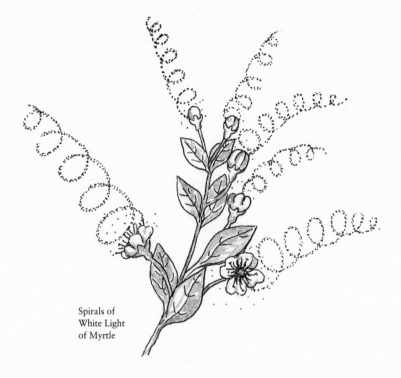

Spirals of
White Light
of Myrtle

Colour signature: Myrtle is a large evergreen bush with brownish-red bark and small scented blue-green pointed leaves. It has fragrant white flowers followed by small blue-black berries. Myrtle was used in ancient Greece as the symbol of love and immortality and the white flowers were thought to symbolise peace. The oil is usually made from the blue-green leaves and twigs, and so carries a turquoise colour signature. The berries also imbue the oil with the indigo ray which harmonises with the third eye centre and associate this oil with intuition, insight and knowledge. The drying qualities of the blue-green ray combats mucus in the lungs and sinuses and its antiseptic and astringent qualities make it a useful component of skin tonics and lotions. Emotionally, Myrtle soothes the emotions and helps refine the senses raising one's awareness and appreciation of beauty and promoting a search for truth.

Level of healing	Aromatherapy	Colour therapy
Physical	good for respiratory tract infections	turquoise to throat and chest
	boosts the immune system	turquoise to thymus and spleen
	urinary problems	indigo to kidneys and bladder
	aphrodisiac qualities	indigo over lower body, or feet
Emotional	soothes feelings of anger, blame, irritation and frustration	green to heart chakra
	moves repressed emotions through verbal expression	blue to throat chakra
	promotes self-love and feeling of value	green to heart chakra
Mental	sedates the lower mind allowing one connection with the higher mind and intuition	blue to brow chakra
	soothing and calming to the anxious mind	blue to crown and solar-plexus
Spiritual	brings insight, understanding and knowledge	indigo to brow chakra
	moves congestion in the subtle bodies	turquoise to whole aura

Precautions: could irritate mucous membranes in high doses.

Affirmations: With the turquoise ray in Myrtle I see truth and beauty in all things.

NEROLI (Orange Blossom)

CITRUS AURANTIUM

Healing colours/s: orange or yellow depending on type
Colour aroma treatment/s: colour massage, colour aroma lamp, spray mist, colour aroma bath, colour compresses
Chakra affinity: sacral, solar-plexus
Life qualities: innovation, flexibility, integrity, simplicity, resolution, connection, sharing

Colour signature: Neroli is made from the twice-yearly blossoms of the Chinese orange-flower tree. It can also be made from the petals of the mandarin and lemon tree, and the colour signature will alter accordingly. Neroli has a beautifully rich floral fragrance which is often used as a perfume in toiletries and sprays. Its orange ray gives it a sedative and soporific effect on the senses and mind, making one feel sleepy and peaceful. Orange has a releasing effect on the emotions, often helping express feelings through the release of tears. Neroli contains the orange ray mixed with white light which is absorbed through the blossoms. This means that Neroli brings lightness and brightness to our lives so we feel both uplifted and joyous but also tranquil and at peace.

Level of healing	Aromatherapy	Colour therapy
Physical	very soothing effect on the sympathetic nervous system	blue on heart
	stimulates sexual desires	orange on sacral area
	cleanses blood and relaxes the heart	blue on heart
	promotes skin elasticity, good for stretch marks, scars and thread veins	orange followed by blue over affected area
	calms the intestines	blue and orange on lower abdomen

Emotional	calming effect on anxious people	orange on sacral chakra
	lifts sorrows and helps us share our pain	orange to solar-plexus and throat chakra
	good for pre-menstrual depression, PMT and menopausal problems	blue on sacral area
Mental	very relaxing to the mind, relieves nervous tension, stress, anxiety, insomnia due to depression	blue on sacral area
Spiritual	regenerative properties, helps reform aura after illness or accident	orange on soles of the feet

Precautions: non-toxic, non-sensitising, non-irritant, may be too relaxing if you need to be alert or undertake mental activity.

Affirmations: With the soothing blue of Neroli, I am able to sleep deeply and wake refreshed.

NIAOULI

MELALEUCA VIRIDIFLORA

Healing colours/s: yellow, violet and turquoise
Colour aroma treatment/s: colour aroma bath, colour massage, colour inhalant, colour breathing, colour aroma lamp, room spray mist
Chakra affinity: heart and crown
Life qualities: clarity, eloquence, spontaneous, sparkling, refreshed, cleansed

Colour signature: Niaouli is a large bushy tree with yellow flowers which is native to Australia. The South Sea Island of New Caledonia has plentiful Niaouli trees to which the islanders have attributed the fact that their island is malaria free. The yellow oil is made from the purple flowering tips of the tree. It is these two colours which imbue Niaouli with strong antiseptic qualities, giving it the therapeutic action of warding off infectious illnesses. The oil also vibrates on the turquoise frequency which is the colour found in the clear aquamarine waters surrounding the islands on which it is found. The culture of South Sea Islanders reveals an open heart centre as they have a loving and sharing attitude to life. The blue and green energy mixture in Niaouli is an excellent oil for boosting the immune system, working and warding off infections and it has a positive and healing effect on the respiratory tract and lungs. The strong Violet ray has pain relieving properties which helps treat burns, while the yellow purifies wounds, boils, cuts and ulcers.

Level of healing	Aromatherapy	Colour therapy
Physical	firms tissues and aids healing	violet followed by turquoise on localised area
	tonic action on the intestines, use against intestinal parasites and urinary infections	violet and turquoise on lower abdomen
	tissue stimulant promotes circulation in localised tissues	violet over affected area
	chest infections, cough, asthma, sinusitis, catarrh, influenza, pneumonia, laryngitis	turquoise over chest and throat
Emotional	refreshing and uplifting to the spirits	violet over solar-plexus
	helps release repressed emotions	turquoise over solar-plexus
Mental	revives and stimulates, refreshes the mind	violet over crown, followed by turquoise
Spiritual	helps with inner communication and deep past life healing	turquoise over crown

Precautions: Possible sensitisation on some people

Affirmations: With the turquoise ray in Niaouli I am building a strong immune system.

NUTMEG

MYRISTICA FRAGRANS
Healing colours/s: orange
Colour aroma treatment/s:, spray mists, colour compresses, colour aromatic cooking, colour aroma lamps, room diffusers, perfumes, colour breathing,
Chakra affinity: sacral
Life qualities: multi-facetedness, vitality, dynamism, grace

Colour signature: This large evergreen tree has smooth grey-brown bark, dense foliage and small yellow flowers. The oil is derived from the kernel of the seed which is a bright orange-brown. The strength of the tree and the hardness of the seed gives qualities of exuberance, vitality and stamina. The orange colour signature gives it a stimulating action on the circulation and digestive system. On an emotional level the orange vibration promotes a loving, animated attitude to relationships which gives a person an aura of love and abundance. Nutmeg has long been used as an aphrodisiac as it is a tonic to the reproductive system, but it also frees us from our reparations and inhibitions so we can celebrate our sexuality. The complementary colour to orange, indigo is also present in nutmeg, acting as a protective force.

Level of healing	Aromatherapy	Colour therapy
Physical	wards off bacterial infection	indigo to soles of feet
	appetite stimulant, stimulates digestion	orange to stomach
	frigidity, impotence	orange to pelvic area
	eases muscular aches and pains	orange light to whole body or feet

Emotional	liberating effect on the emotions	orange to sacral chakra
	warming and releasing feelings of guilt or dejection	orange to sacral chakra
Mental	reviving to the mind improves nervous fatigue	orange to solar-plexus
	lifts depression	orange to sacral centre
	exhilarating and activates the mind	orange to solar-plexus
Spiritual	protection	indigo to whole body, colour breathing
	helps addictions, especially drug-related by releasing childhood trauma	orange to sacral chakra
	bringer of prosperity and abundance	orange to sacral chakra

Precautions: Avoid during pregnancy. Use in small doses as it can be toxic and hallucinogenic.

Affirmations: With nutmeg, the orange ray makes me sparkling, joyous and dynamic.

ORANGE
CITRUS DULCIS (sweet orange), CITURS VULGARIS/SINENSIS
Healing colours/s: orange
Colour aroma treatment/s: solarised drink or food, colour aroma bath, colour massage, colour skin tonic and lotion, aroma candles, room diffusers
Chakra affinity: sacral
Life qualities: happy, positive, out-going, joyous, strong, courageous, creative

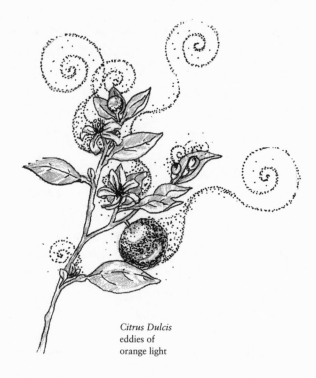

Citrus Dulcis
eddies of
orange light

Colour signature: Orange essential oil is made from the peel of the sweet or bitter orange, hence its colour affinity. Like other orange ray oils it has a grounding, stimulating and releasing action. Its most important quality is its ability to lift depression and bring joy into our lives. On a physical level the colour orange boosts the immune system, and it is well known that orange fruit and vegetables contain beta-carotene which fight off anti-oxidants in our system. Orange is therefore an excellent tonic, helping ward off disease and aiding the absorption of Vitamin C. Emotionally orange has a releasing effect, instilling us with courage and opening creative channels. The earth connection of Orange helps us relax and enhances physical enjoyment, so that we become sensual, warm and physically expressive. Some people have a strong dislike for orange or citrus aromas in general and it is likely they have a strong association with citrus growing countries, especially in the Mediterranean in this or a previous life.

Level of healing	Aromatherapy	Colour therapy
Physical	brings down high levels of cholesterol	orange over the soles of the feet
	helps form collagen for repair of body tissues	orange over soles of the feet
	good for gastric complaints, calms the stomach	orange over the chest
	opens chest, use to improve breathing for chronic asthma, bronchitis	orange over stomach
	stimulates bile aiding digestion of fats	orange and yellow over liver
Emotional	anti-depressant, helps stimulate you when feeling bored, good for selfishness and stubbornness	orange over sacral chakra
Mental	lifts depression, dispels tension and stress releases addictions	orange over the sacral chakra
Spiritual	charges and revitalises the aura	orange irradiation of the whole body

Precautions: may irritate a sensitive skin, can also be photo-toxic with high doses.

Affirmations: I radiate energy and vitality with the orange ray.

OREGANO

ORIGANUM VULGARE

Healing colours/s: green and pale-yellow
Colour aroma treatment/s: colour aroma bath, colour massage, colour room diffuser, colour compresses, colour gemstones
Chakra affinity: heart and solar-plexus
Life qualities: calmness, self-reliance, balance, kindness, tolerance, sympathy

Colour signature: This bushy herb has dark green oval leaves and the flowers are formed in clusters which are grey-white. The Greek word for Origanum means 'joy of the mountains' which is reflected in its uplifting green and yellow energy. The yellow ray found in Origanum, purifies the liver and gently warms the circulation. The fresh herbaceous aroma is gently warming, uplifting and soothing to the nervous and respiratory system. This makes it a wonderful oil for the treatment of stress and for its pacifying but refreshing qualities. The ability of Origanum to bring relaxation to the mind allows the yellow energy to flow releasing the deep-seated fears. Its historical use by monks for celibacy is reflected in its ability to balance the emotions and to bring a feeling of inner wholeness and stillness.

Level of healing	Aromatherapy	Colour therapy
Physical	reduces sexual drive	green to lower body
	acute asthma, coughs, bronchitis	green to chest
	constipation, colic, flatulence	green to stomach, liver
	eases stiff joints, muscular pain, strains and rheumatics	green to soles of the feet or affected area
Emotional	brings emotional comfort in times of grief, rejection, loneliness	green to heart chakra
	releases anger, anxiety, irritability	green to heart chakra
	calms and balances emotions, good for hysteria	green to heart chakra

Mental	headaches, migraines, delirium, phobias, insomnia	green to back of head or temples
	mental tiredness caused by stress	green to back of head
	releases fears of the mind	green to top of head
Spiritual	strengthens ability to withdraw from the world	green to crown chakra
	provides spiritual focus and calmness	green to brow chakra

Precautions: Avoid during pregnancy.

Affirmations: With the green ray in Origanum I find inner balance and strength.

PALMAROSA

CYMBOPOGON MARTINI

Healing colours/s: pink and green
Colour aroma treatment/s: colour baths, colour massage, colour creams and lotions, colour room diffuser, colour spray mist, perfumes, colour candles
Chakra affinity: Heart
Life qualities: healing, flexible, relaxed, harmonious, peaceful, nurturing, loving

Colour signature: Palmarosa is distilled from a tall slender grass which has a geranium-like scent and which is dried before it flowers. Palmarosa is a truly feminine oil and its pink colour signature has a strong affinity with the heart chakra. It has the ability to harmonise the feminine aspect in both sexes and to calm and soothe the emotions as well as restore balance in the body. Its natural harmonising qualities make it excellent for skincare and maintaining water balance and a constant healthy appetite. Most grasses are in sympathetic resonance with the colour green and this gives them the healing property of encouraging healthy cell growth and regeneration.

Green is the colour which relates to the heart and the ability to feel free especially at times when we feel emotionally restricted. Together with the flexibility and movement indicated by the grass itself, Palmarosa oil allows us physical and emotional space to move and grow.

Level of healing	Aromatherapy	Colour therapy
Physical	reduces temperature and fevers	green light over heart
	a tonic to the digestive system and stomach	green light over stomach
	restores water balance	green light on pituitary gland or corresponding foot reflex
	hydrating to the skin	pink to affected area
	aids cell regeneration	green light over appropriate area
Emotional	gently uplifting and soothing to the emotions, heals with love	pink and green over heart chakra
	softens a hard heart with love	pink to heart chakra
Mental	clearing and uplifting to the mind	green to the back of the head
	heals nervous exhaustion and stress	green to the crown chakra
Spiritual	Brings a feeling of freedom of movement in your life	pink over the heart chakra

Precautions: None known.

Affirmations: With the green ray, Palmarosa gives me freedom to express myself.
The pink ray in Palmarosa fills my whole being with love and light.

PARSLEY

Petroselinium sativum
Healing colours/s: green and yellow
Colour aroma treatment/s: perfumes, colour aroma bath, colour room
diffuser, colour breathing and meditation, colour aroma cooking
Chakra affinity: heart and solar-plexus
Life qualities: caring, compassion, calmness, stillness, forgiveness

Colour signature: This well known herb has bright green crinkled foliage with green-yellow flowers and small green-brown seeds. The essential oil is a yellow or amber coloured liquid giving parsley seed oil the healing qualities of both green and yellow energy. Looking at the plant with its soft curling leaves and love of moisture, we can see how it relates to healing through the emotions which are related to the water element. Parsley promotes a soft, caring attitude opening the heart to nature and allowing us to find forgiveness through compassion and love. The yellow ray in parsley has a cleansing and purifying action on the body and together they give our life a boost, making room for love to flow. Parsley has a diuretic action which removes toxins from the blood. The yellow ray also helps clear repressed emotions and is calming and refreshing to the mind.

Level of healing	Aromatherapy	Colour therapy
Physical	cleanses kidneys and bladder	green to kidneys
	balances menstrual difficulties	green to pelvis
	cleanses digestive system and good for indigestion, colic and has a laxative action	yellow to stomach
	freshens breath	green to throat
Emotional	harmonises emotions by releasing envy, greed, jealousy and resentment helping us to forgive	green to the heart chakra
	opens the heart to nature	green to the heart chakra
	promotes compassion and empathy through communication	green to the heart chakra

Mental	gives you space to think	green to the back of the head
	calming and relaxing to the mind	green to the pituitary gland
Spiritual	refreshing to the soul, through stillness	green to the whole body
	allows time for new beginnings	green to the heart chakra
	inner healing and peace	green to the heart chakra

Precautions: Avoid during pregnancy, use in moderation as can be an irritant and moderately toxic.

Affirmations: With the healing green in Parsley, I reach out with love and compassion to all living things.

PATCHOULI
POGOSTEMOM PATCHOULI
Healing colours/s: orange, violet, (some oils yellow)
Colour aroma treatment/s: colour aroma massage, colour bath, perfume, colour aroma skincare treatments, colour aroma lamp, spray mists, aromatic candles, meditation
Chakra affinity: sacral, solar-plexus, crown
Life qualities: grounded, decisive, expansive, assured, witty, lucid, astute

Colour signature: Patchouli takes its colour signature from the dark orange colour of the oil which is distilled from the white flowers which have a purple hue. Patchouli oil has the tonic affect of orange especially on the libido and its releasing qualities promote the flow of creative expression. It is a wonderful anti-depressant and has a bracing effect on the nervous system. The orange/yellow energy acts as a diuretic releasing water from the system and then maintains water balance by the action of the violet ray on the endocrine system. The violet ray in Patchouli gives its astringent and fungicidal properties. By working through the endocrine system appetite is curbed and sweating produced. Violet energy is a tissue regenerator, and Patchouli oil has been known for centuries to cool inflamed conditions especially a dry, hot skin. The mixture of blue and red contained in the violet activates new cell growth but at the same time exerts a healing and balancing action.

Level of healing	Aromatherapy	Colour therapy
Physical	sores, wounds, eczema, chapped, dry and tired skin insect repellent	orange and violet light to affected area, spray mist, room diffuser
	frigidity, creative expression through the body	orange to pelvis
	water retention, obesity, cellulite, appetite suppressant	yellow/violet to crown or pituitary reflex on foot
Emotional	balances mood swings	violet to pituitary gland
	tonic for tired spirits, nervous exhaustion, helps the weak willed, apprehension, anxiety	orange, yellow to solar-plexus
	grounding and promotes security	red to base chakra
Mental	banished negative thoughts, stress anti-depressive, helps decision-making	violet to crown orange to solar-plexus
Spiritual	integrates base and crown chakras	red to base, violet to crown
	brings well-being and contentment	orange to soles of feet, violet to crown

Precautions: None known.

Affirmations: Patchouli oil brings me the orange ray of positivity and contentment. The violet light in patchouli helps my body find its own balance. Annoint your wrist or temples with a drop of oil before saying these affirmations.

PETITGRAIN

CITRUS VULGARIS/AURANTIUM
Healing colours/s: green, pale yellow
Colour aroma treatment/s: colour aroma baths, inhalers, colour massages, colour aroma room diffusers, spray mists and perfumes, colour breathing, candles
Chakra affinity: heart, solar-plexus
Life qualities: balanced, optimistic, expressive, relaxed, refreshed

Colour signature: This oil is made from the leaves and young shoots of the orange tree, and is a pale yellow liquid with a fresh floral citrus scent. Its affinity with the green ray gives it a sedating and soothing healing quality which is especially relaxing to the heart. Relaxation is brought about by easing of breathing, while the pale yellow energy works on the nervous system, refreshing and reviving the body. The yellow ray helps the green energy to pervade through all the subtle bodies making Petitgrain an excellent oil for use during convalescence. Petitgrain is a refreshing and uplifting oil which fills us with inner strength and optimism helping us seek new opportunities and open ourselves to love.

Level of healing	Aromatherapy	Colour therapy
Physical	relaxes muscle spasms	green over affected area
	calms stomach and digestion	green over stomach
	cleansing and toning to the skin	green over liver, gallbladder

Emotional	soothing to the emotions by sedating the nervous system	green over the heart chakra
	calms anger and panic, good for all stress	green over the heart chakra
	allows us space and time for inner healing	green over the heart chakra
Mental	refreshing to the mind calms racing thoughts and promotes inner communication with the heart	green to the pituitary gland
	good for insomnia	green over the back of the head
Spiritual	revitalises the spirit	green over the crown chakra
	balances and restores the energy in the aura	green light to the whole body
	fills one with inner strength and awareness of divine love	yellow to the solar-plexus

Precautions: None known.

Affirmations: With the green ray in Petitgrain I am relaxed and balanced and optimistic about the future.

PIMENTO
PIMENTA OFFICINALIS
Healing colours/s: indigo and orange
Colour aroma treatment/s: room diffuser, aroma bath (check for sensitivity first), gemstone healing, colour candle
Chakra affinity: sacral and brow
Life qualities: expression, openness, self-esteem, inner security, involvement

Colour signature: This evergreen tree produces two kidney-shaped green seeds which turn glossy blue-black when they mature. The liquid made by distilling the seeds divides into two separate parts and when mixed together creates the essential oil, which is a yellowish-red or brown colour. Pimento oil, therefore, contains a balance of the two colours, orange and indigo. The orange ray gives it a warming and releasing character, while the indigo ray opens the brow centre, allowing insight and understanding of relationships and life situations. By working in harmony, the orange and blue help us release repressed emotions through openness and self-expression. The deepness of the blue heals the causal body and allows us to bring insight and clarity into our affairs, so that we can value ourselves and build up a more positive self-image. Pimento is a good overall tonic and antidepressant and its orange colour signature harmonises with the digestive system.

Level of healing	Aromatherapy	Colour therapy
Physical	warms chills, coughs, colds, bronchitis, powerfully analgesic	orange over chest and throat
	helps stiffness of the joints and rheumatism	orange to feet or affected area
	good for nausea	orange to liver
	relieves headaches and toothache	indigo to throat and temples
Emotional	warming and releasing to the emotions	orange to sacral chakra
	promotes sharing and communication	orange to sacral chakra
	helps us live in the moment	orange to sacral chakra
Mental	lifts depression	orange to brow
	nervous exhaustion and mental stress	orange to solar-plexus
	releases restrictive mind patterns	indigo to brow

Spiritual   clarity of vision   indigo to brow
            intuitive responses to   indigo to crown
            relationships so you know what
            is right
             deep healing for a shock
            situation

Precautions: can cause skin irritation, use in low dilution as this oil can irritate mucous membranes.

Affirmations: With the balancing colours in Indigo I connect with my creativity and know that all will be well.

PEPPERMINT
MENTHA PIPERITA
Healing colours/s: green and violet
Colour aroma treatment/s: colour baths, colour aroma massage, room diffuser, spray mists, colour breathing, solar-charged food and drink, gemstone healing,
Chakra affinity: heart and crown
Life qualities: expansion, freshness, exhilaration, renewal, awakening, lucidity

Colour signature: This well-known green herb loves damp conditions. 'White' Peppermint has green stems and leaves, but the 'black' peppermint has dark green leaves and purplish stems with red-violet flowers. Water is the element associated with the emotions and the green energy in Peppermint is excellent for the treatment of shock, stress and nervous tension. Green energy has an affinity with the digestive system as well as having a positive effect on the respiration. It relaxes the heart muscles and sympathetic nervous system, thus having a calming and sedating effect on us. Although penetrating in its aroma, Peppermint has a cooling and healing effect and helps relieve pain. Its penetrating action stimulates the mind aiding concentration and sharpness when we need to be alert and it has an uplifting action on the emotions. Both red and violet energy stimulate and detoxify the kidneys thus encouraging the flow of life-force energy through the chakra system.

Level of healing	Aromatherapy	Colour therapy
Physical	cooling action on the skin, acne, scabies, toothache, dermatitis	green on affected area
	muscular pain, palpitations	green over heart and affected area
	bronchitis, sinusitis, asthma, catarrh	green over chest
	detoxifies the liver, good for nausea, flatulence, cramp, colic, dyspepsia	green over liver
	colds, flu and fevers	green light to feet, followed by violet
Emotional	uplifting and gently warming	green to heart chakra
	helps self-acceptance and space to be yourself	green to heart chakra
	expansive, allowing freshness of spirit	green to heart chakra
Mental	stress, migraine, vertigo, fainting	green to head or feet
	invigorating allowing us to see life from a different point of view	green to the crown chakra
Spiritual	stimulates the flow of energy between heart and crown	green to whole body, gemstone healing, colour breathing
	cleanses and balances the aura	green to heart chakra

Precautions: Use in moderation, can irritate sensitive skin.

Affirmations: Peppermint allows me to feel fresh and ready for a new day.

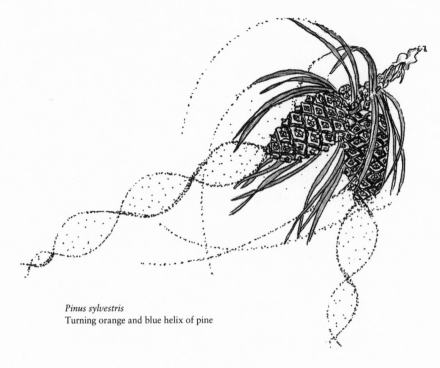

Pinus sylvestris
Turning orange and blue helix of pine

PINE

PINUS SYLVESTRIS
Healing colours/s: orange and blue
Colour aroma treatment/s: colour massage, spray mist, colour aroma
bath, colour aroma breathing
Chakra affinity: sacral
Life qualities: acceptance of love, sharing, self-worth, patience,
understanding

Colour signature: At first, one may think that the Scotch Pine has resonance
with the green ray, but the oil takes its main colour signature from its
reddish-brown bark and its orange-yellow flowers. Orange energy gives
us direction and perseverance while the green gives us physical and
emotional space to pursue our destiny. The warming, expanding and
releasing qualities of orange make the Scotch Pine ideal for the treatment
of bronchial catarrh, asthma, and blocked sinuses. Its gentle warming action
soothes a sore throat while its complementary blue ray also gives it an
anti-viral and antiseptic action. So while Scotch Pine warms and soothes,
it also heals and disinfects. It provides a good tonic for the mind, especially

when one is tired and suffering from mental fatigue. Pine allows us to develop a more positive self-image, and this self-confidence helps you make changes in your life.

Level of healing	Aromatherapy	Colour therapy
Physical	normalises blood pressure and reduces heat use for excessive perspiration and the treatment of fleas and lice	green light or scarf to the head
	arthritis, gout, rheumatism, poor circulation	orange to the feet and base of spine
	stimulates adrenals	orange to base and kidneys
	heals cuts and skin irritations like eczema and psoriasis	green bandages or solarised oil to affected parts
Emotional	nervous exhaustion, stress related conditions	green light to solar-plexus
	builds self-love and teaches forgiveness	green to heart chakra
	builds self-confidence by moving repressed emotions of guilt and rejection	orange to sacral centre
Mental	exhilarating to the mind so use for general mental fatigue	blue light irradiation to head
Spiritual	restorative and cleansing to the aura	blue light irradiation to whole body

Precautions: non-toxic, non-irritant except on sensitive skins.

Affirmations: With the aromatic Pine I can breathe more deeply and easily. The orange ray renews my energy and strength.

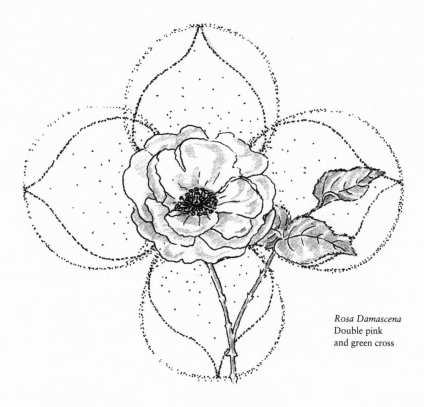

Rosa Damascena
Double pink
and green cross

ROSE

ROSA DAMASCENA

Healing colours/s: pink and green
Colour aroma treatment/s: colour baths, solarised lotions, colour toilet
waters, perfumes, colour massage, colour aroma lamps, colour breathing
Chakra affinity: heart
Life qualities: unconditional love, radiance, gentleness, caring,
gracefulness, humility

Colour signature: The Damask rose is small prickly shrub which has an
abundance of highly fragrant pink blooms on whitish hairy leaves. The
rose has always been associated with love and especially femininity. Its
sympathetic pink vibration works on balancing the feminine aspect within
both sexes and helps many female ailments. The pink colour energy in
Rose helps transform passion to compassion and selfish love to selfless love.
The green energy permeates the parasympathetic nervous system to calm,
balance and heal. Rose Otto is steam distilled and the oil balances

circulation, relaxes the heart, and is excellent in the treatment of shock and stress. The pink ray in Rose Otto brings with it a feeling of restfulness through acceptance of ourselves and the knowledge that we do not need to prove anything to the world.

Level of healing	Aromatherapy	Colour therapy
Physical	broken capillaries, dry skin, eczema, herpes, mature/sensitive complexion	colour charged lotions, creams, oils for massage
	Balances blood pressure and promotes the circulation	pink/green over the heart for 5 minutes each colour
	Soothing for asthma, coughs, hay fever	green light over chest and throat
	Clears liver and helps nausea aphrodisiac and benefits all female organs, balances menstrual cycle, uterine disorders	green light over liver pink light over pelvis area
Emotional	promotes a feeling of well-being and happiness, Soothes and uplifts the emotions, PMS, grieving	pink scarf or light over the heart
	appreciation of beauty through an open heart	pink to heart chakra
Mental	helps mental fatigue, exhaustion and stress	green scarf over the back of the head
	helps retention and memory	pink to crown chakra
Spiritual	allowing unconditional love to flow	pink gemstone or wearing pink over heart

Precautions: Avoid during pregnancy. Rose Otto is a highly potent oil so do not use in cases of high blood pressure or epilepsy.

Affirmations: When pink is flowing through me I feel happy and positive about myself. Pink light shows me that I am able to give and receive love unconditionally.

ROSE
ROSA CENTIFOLIA
Healing colours/s: red, deep pink
Colour aroma treatment/s: colour massage, colour bath, colour toilet water, solarised creams and lotions, perfume, colour aroma lamps, meditation, soaps
Chakra affinity: base and heart
Life qualities: harmonious, reassuring, comforting, inner vitality, giving, loving

Colour signature: Different roses have different special qualities imbued into them through the colour energy in the petals of the flowers. The cabbage rose has a mass of pink or rosy-purple flowers, which reinforces its use as an aphrodisiac. The purple energy these flowers contain, works as a narcotic which relaxes the mind. The oil from the Cabbage rose is obtained by solvent extraction and is deeper in colouring and rich in vital life-force energy. The red colour vibration in this oil makes it excellent for helping the emotions to flow, thus aiding our ability to give of ourselves. Impotence and frigidity can be helped in this way. The mixed colour signature of pink and green of the Damask rose gives us grounding and confidence in ourselves but allows us to connect with our higher nature so that we can allow creative energy to flow through us. All rose oils have antiseptic qualities and are particular beneficial to the skin, allowing the radiance of the soul to shine through so we glow with good health.

Level of healing	Aromatherapy	Colour therapy
Physical	soothing, compresses to reduce swelling and inflammation, good for the eyes	pink to the eyes and affected area
	tonic to the heart, stomach and liver, uterus	pink to the heart and stomach, liver
	aphrodisiac	red to base of the spine
	mild astringent and antiseptic	pink to affected area
	healing balm for the skin and for pain relief	pink to affected area
Emotional	comforting and reassuring to the emotions	pink to heart chakra
	opens the heart to divine love	red to heart chakra
Mental	balances the psyche in cases of addictions and shock, also amnesia	pink to crown chakra
	anti-depressant and for mental fatigue	red to solar-plexus chakra
Spiritual	uplifting to the spirit, union with the divine, fulfilment	pink to whole body
	cleansing and transmuting the energy in the aura	pink light over the heart

Precautions: non-toxic, non-irritant, non-sensitising.

Affirmations: The deep pink ray runs through my system bringing me divine love. With the deep pink light I release all my past pain, and feel calm and free.

ROSEWOOD

ANIBA ROSAEODORA

Healing colours/s: pink and green
Colour aroma treatment/s: colour baths, colour massage, room
diffusers, spray mist, skin lotions, colour candles, colour breathing
Chakra affinity: heart
Life qualities: benevolence, tolerance, comfort, reliability, constancy

Colour signature: This lovely soothing oil is made from the 'heartwood'
of this tropical evergreen tree. Rosewood has reddish bark and yellow
flowers, and the essential oil has a fragrant sweet woody aroma. Like all
trees, the Rosewood has a strengthening effect especially when one feels
overburdened with worries and problems. The green and pink energy of
this tree opens the heart chakra making it a lovely oil for emotional
balance and the treatment of stress. It gives comfort to those who have
suffered emotional or physical abuse and helps them recover their sexual
desires. It is mild and safe for use in skin care products and helps with
sexual problems due to nervous tension and stress. In order to preserve
this rare tree, it is better to substitute another pink and green oil like
Geranium or Rose damascena.

Level of healing	Aromatherapy	Colour therapy
Physical	boosting immune system generally where suffering from chronic illness	pink over the kidneys, green over the thymus
	boosting libido where sexual drive is low	pink over pelvis and heart
	skin and tissue regenerator and good for cuts and wounds	green over affected area
Emotional	Overall balancing effect on the emotions especially mood swings, soothing and relaxing	pink and green over heart chakra
	brings maturity through stability and constancy	pink followed by green to heart chakra

Mental	balancing effect on the mind by stabilising central nervous system, promotes empathy, open-mindedness and tolerance	green over the crown chakra green to heart chakra
Spiritual	balancing the energy in the aura	pink light on the feet, green light on the crown

Precautions: non-toxic, non-irritant, non-sensitising

Affirmations: With the green ray there is harmony in my body and mind. Pink energy allows my emotions to heal naturally in their own time.

ROSEMARY
ROSMARINUS OFFICINALIS
Healing colours/s: blue
Colour aroma treatment/s: colour aroma bath, hair rinse, colour aroma lamp, colour aroma massage, colour breathing and inhaling, gemstone healing
Chakra affinity: throat, brow
Life qualities: perception, clarity of vision, intuitive, gracious, loyal

Colour signature: The pale blue flowers of this shrubby evergreen bush gives Rosemary its blue colour signature. The pale blue flowers together with the silvery-green of the leaves indicates a fast vibration of light energy belonging to a high octave of colour. The force-field of blue-violet light produced by Rosemary confirms its reputation from ancient times as a psychic protector and as an aid to developing inner vision. Like all blue vibrations, Rosemary has antiseptic and astringent properties and it has sympathetic resonance with the throat, eyes, ears and head. Its cooling and soothing action makes it wonderful for treatment of mental fatigue, nervous exhaustion and stress-related disorders. The blue ray reflected in the oil is a bringer of high ideals, and a desire for truth, loyalty and justice.

212

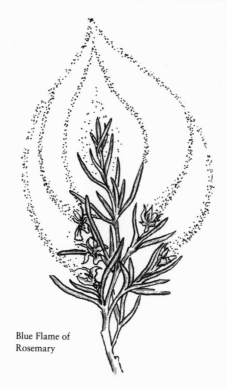

Blue Flame of
Rosemary

Level of healing	Aromatherapy	Colour therapy
Physical	muscular aches and pains poor circulation, rheumatism	blue over legs and hands
	varicose veins	blue over legs
	stimulates the scalp promotes hair growth	blue over head
	hepatitis and jaundice	blue over liver
	asthma, bronchitis, whooping cough	blue over chest
Emotional	helps vocalise thoughts and feelings, purifies the emotions bringing upliftment	blue to throat chakra
	tunes in to one's higher emotions and intuition	blue to throat chakra
	purifies the emotions, bringing upliftment	blue to throat and sacral chakra

Mental	restorative to the mind, headaches due to hypotension	blue to brow chakra
	mental fatigue and nervous exhaustion	blue to brow chakra
	releasing negative mind patterns	blue to brow chakra
Spiritual	psychic protection against negative forces	blue to whole aura
	helps develop sensitivity to subtle forces and higher realms	blue to brow (blue gemstone, or crystal)

Precautions: Do not use during pregnancy, or if you suffer from high blood pressure or epilepsy.

Affirmations: With the pale blue of Rosemary I am in touch with the truth.

SANDALWOOD
SANTALUM ALBUM
Healing colours/s: violet and yellow
Colour aroma treatment/s: solar-charged lotions and creams, perfumes, spray mists, colour baths, colour massage, colour bandages, compresses and poultices, incense and meditation, aromatic colour candles, soaps
Chakra affinity: throat and sacral
Life qualities: connection, peace, unity, serenity, rejuvenation

Colour signature: This small evergreen parasitic tree has a brown-grey trunk, red or pinky-purple flowers and yellowish wood. The oil is made from the heartwood and contains yellow and violet energy. Sandalwood has sympathetic resonance with both these complementary colours for it is both a tonic and a sedative and therefore very special oil. Sandalwood has strong associations with ceremony, serenity and wisdom and is well-known for its use in India as an aid to meditation for it relaxes and sedates the mind. It was also widely used in embalming because of its beneficial action on the skin. The coolness of the violet action soothes and softens the skin especially when infected or itchy. The yellow ray in the oil warms and comforts through a feeling of euphoria and relaxation, while the violet ray purifies at a deep level bringing peace and serenity. The violet ray also gives it aphrodisiac qualities not by stimulation like the warm colour vibrations, but by the cleansing action on the sexual organs. The affinity Sandalwood has with Rose makes it both a good tonic and sedative for the heart.

Level of healing	Aromatherapy	Colour therapy
Physical	bronchitis, coughs, sore throat, laryngitis, chest infections	violet to throat and chest
	nausea, diarrhoea, cystitis	violet to stomach and pelvis
	itchy cracked skin	blue to affected area
	purifies the sexual organs, clears energy blocks causing frigidity and impotence	red to lower abdomen
Emotional	soothes aggression, helps rejection, worthlessness, breakdown	violet to heart and throat
Mental	mental stress, obsession, phobias, relaxing, aids sleep	violet to crown, colour breathing
Spiritual	balances the base and crown chakras	red to base, violet to crown
	helps relax the conscious mind for meditation	violet to crown, meditation

Precautions: In some cases can be toxic. Can cause drowsiness.

Affirmations: With the colour blue ray in Sandalwood I cleanse all negative vibrations from my system. The blue ray is keeping my skin youthful and supple.

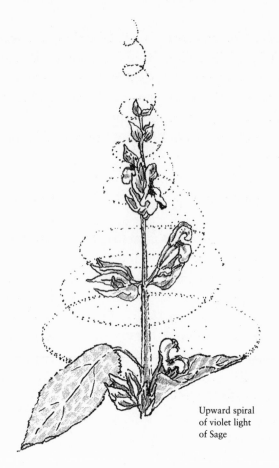

Upward spiral
of violet light
of Sage

SAGE (Spanish)

Salvia lavandulaefolia

Healing colours/s: violet (red and blue), blue
Colour aroma treatment/s: Room diffuser, colour bath, colour massage,
solarised drink, colour aroma lamps, colour breathing, aroma
colour cooking
Chakra affinity: throat, brow,crown
Life qualities: awareness, wisdom, grace, longevity, integrity

Colour signature: Sage is an attractive herb with pretty purple-green leaves
and blue flowers, although there are many different varieties. Sage has
always been associated with wisdom and 'longevity' and was popular in
the middle ages as a tonic and stimulant. Its purple and blue characteristic makes it a Yin oil, and its stimulating qualities come through the mind

and central nervous system rather than through the blood stream. The violet ray works on the body's metabolic processes, controlling the production and flow of hormones. Sage has constricting qualities of Yin energy, and so it arrests bleeding and stimulates the formation of scar tissue. Sage has the cleansing action of violet working through the kidneys, while the red vibration in the oil gently raises blood pressure without stressing the heart. It also has the pain-relieving qualities of blue-violet. The vibrations of Sage give it the ability to balance the crown and base chakra developing our self-awareness so we can walk our true path in life.

Level of healing	Aromatherapy	Colour therapy
Physical	cleansing and purifying to the skin, also for sores and gum infections. Use in cases of excessive sweating, arthritis, rheumatism, jaundice, fluid retention, poor circulation, tonic for digestive system.	blue light over the affected area violet to kidneys and legs and soles of feet violet to the pituitary gland and liver violet to abdomen, stomach
Emotional	Affects the emotions through hormonal balance calms nerves, tiredness, and grief, works on the parasympathetic nervous system.	blue to pituitary gland blue to the heart chakra
Mental	A nerve tonic, good for nervous exhaustion, headaches, stress, depression	blue light to the throat and pituitary gland
Spiritual	brings wisdom, inner knowledge and a seeker of truth purifies and cleanses the aura, thus promoting a long healthy life	violet to crown chakra blue to the third eye and soles of the feet

Precautions: Avoid during pregnancy. In large doses can have an adverse effect on the central nervous system.

Affirmations: With the violet ray my whole system is cleansed and purified. The blue ray heals my wound and is making new cell tissue grow.

STAR ANISE
ILLICIUM VERUM
Healing colours/s: green
Colour aroma treatment/s: spray mists, colour compresses, colour aromatic cooking, colour aroma lamps, room diffusers, perfumes, colour breathing
Chakra affinity: heart, solar-plexus
Life qualities: balance, compassion, natural connection, openness

Colour signature: Star Anise is sometimes known as 'Anise Vert' from the green colouring of the oil which is derived from the green fruits of this evergreen tree. The balancing and loving green energy contained in Star Anise opens the heart centre, helping us to love nature and all living things. The star shapes of the seeds promote our connection with universal forces of the stars and planets allowing us the freedom to explore our spiritual connections. On a physical level, the green ray has a therapeutic action on the digestion and Star Anise is a well-known aperitif and stomachic which also has a carminative and diuretic action. It balances the metabolism through its action on the pituitary gland. Emotionally it is a very cleansing oil, bringing us universal love and peace.

Level of healing	Aromatherapy	Colour therapy
Physical	warming to the respiratory system	yellow to chest
	soothes sore throats and chests	green to chest
	regulates menstruation	green to pelvis
	healing to infections	green to soles of the feet

Emotional	soothing and healing to the emotions	green to the heart chakra
	regulates eating disorders by balancing the pituitary and building self-love	green to the pituitary and brown chakra
	gently stimulating but calming to the mind	green colour breathing
Mental	allows one to see things in a balanced way	green to crown chakra
	freeing restrictive thoughts	green colour breathing and inhalation
	connection to the natural forces	green to the heart chakra
Spiritual	opens the crown chakra through universal love	green to the heart chakra

Precautions: Can over-stimulate the nervous system, and allergy suffers should not use it.

Affirmations: Star-anise helps me regain balance and harmony in my body and mind.

TEA TREE
Melaleuca alternifolia
Healing colours/s: indigo and yellow
Colour aroma treatment/s: colour soaps, toothpaste, solarised gargle, spray mists, room diffusers, colour breathing and inhaling, solarised water or tea
Chakra affinity: third eye and crown
Life qualities: visionary, purity, sensibility, imaginative, perceptive

Colour signature: Tea-tree is a small Australian tree or shrub with needle-like leaves and heads of purplish yellow flowers. It was used by Aboriginal people for thousands of years to protect them from illness and to ward off evil spirits and was adopted by the early settlers to make a fortifying drink. The oil is made from the leaves and twigs and is a strong cleanser and healer. As Tea-tree is a very powerful immune-stimulant it is especially useful for warding off bacterial and fungal infection, and all types of viruses. The indigo ray which is strongly present has an anti-bacterial, anti-viral and antiseptic action on our system. Tea Tree opens the brow chakra allowing us to go beyond the conscious mind. It helps us release our fears and anxieties and to trust in the higher guidance which we can receive from our inner voice, especially when revealed to us in dreams.

Level of healing	Aromatherapy	Colour therapy
Physical	respiratory tract infections, coughs, sinusitis, asthma, tuberculosis, whooping cough	indigo to chest and throat
	thrush, vaginitis, cystitis, sores, blisters, verrucas, warts, mouth ulcers	indigo to pelvis area indigo gargle or applied to affected area
	colds, flu, infectious illnesses	indigo to chest
Emotional	hypochondria, fear of illness or dying, shock, hysteria	indigo to third eye
	encourages idealism and higher emotions	indigo to brow chakra
Mental	sedative to the mind, hypnotic	indigo to crown
Spiritual	purges the aura of harmful vibrations and dissolves negativity before it reaches the subtle bodies	indigo to whole body, crystal to brow
	psychic protection	indigo to third eye

Precautions: non-toxic, non irritant, use with care on sensitive skins

Affirmations: With Tea-tree I am safe and protected from all harm. The indigo ray strengthens my immune system so I can fight off illness.

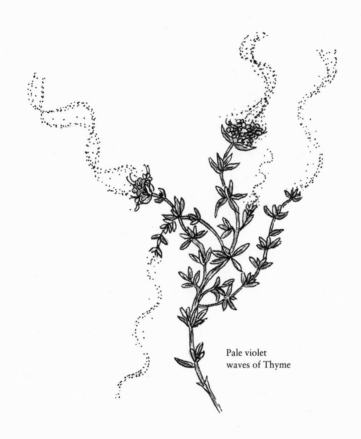

Pale violet
waves of Thyme

THYME (RED)

Thymus vulgaris

Healing colours/s: red and green
Colour aroma treatment/s: colour breathing, solar charged gargle,
colour poultice, aroma handkerchief, colour aroma bath (morning only)
Chakra affinity: base and heart
Life qualities: focused, tolerant, helpful, balanced, quietly confident

Colour signature: Red thyme belongs to the thyme family which are perennial evergreen small shrubs, with grey-green leaves and pale purple, pink or white flowers. The Colour signature of the Red thyme is taken from the red or orange-brown liquid produced which has a powerful spicy aroma. Red energy opens the base chakra flooding our system with warming earth energy which makes us active and outgoing. This energy is useful when we lack direction, as it makes us more focused and gives us stamina to walk firmly on our path in life. The supportive and fortifying nature of Thyme is gently empowering, assisting us to overcome physical and mental exhaustion. Red Thyme, like its colour signature, is useful for stimulating circulation by strengthening the action of the kidneys, helpful in cases of obesity and cellulitis, gout, and muscular aches and pains. Its affinity with red also attracts the healing qualities of green, and so it can be used to treat the respiratory system and to balance the masculine and feminine energy within us.

Level of healing	Aromatherapy	Colour therapy
Physical	use in mouthwashes and gargles for catarrh, coughs, laryngitis, sinusitis, sore throat, tonsillitis	green light therapy on the chest and throat to cool the system and treat inflamed bronchi and throat
	boosts the immune system, strengthening the production of red blood cells. Low blood pressure, coldness and chills	red light therapy to the soles of the feet and to base chakra
Emotional	revives low spirits, depression	red over the soles of the feet
	counteracts shyness and introversion	red over base chakra
Mental	aids memory and concentration, mental exhaustion, releases mental blocks and trauma	red light over the base chakra

Spiritual	helps us find purpose in life	red to base chakra
	grounding and helps us connect to the everyday world	red to base chakra
	strengthens the life force energy in the aura	red light over the soles of the feet and base chakra

Precautions: Avoid in pregnancy, use in moderation and low dosage, and do not use in cases of high blood pressure.

Affirmations: With the red ray I feel secure, safe and warm. My system is strengthened and protected against infection with the red ray.

VERBENA
LIPPIA CITRIODORA
Healing colours/s: green and pink
Colour aroma treatment/s: colour baths, colour massage, spray mists and lotions, colour compresses, colour aromatic cooking, colour aroma lamps, room diffusers, perfumes, colour breathing,
Chakra affinity: heart
Life qualities: gentleness, balance, sensitivity, giving, forgiving

Colour signature: This small ornamental shrub has very fragrant delicate light green leaves with pale pink flowers. The oil is made from the scented leaves and contains the strong healing green colour signature, reinforced by the pink ray revealed in its flowers. The relaxing and refreshing qualities of green works through the parasympathetic nervous system, promoting deep breathing and calming and soothing the mind. Verbena vibrates on the green ray, the colour associated with the heart chakra, and its harmonising aroma helps us relax and release our anxieties and worries. The cleansing action helps us clear out emotional baggage. The green ray is able to offer us physical and emotional space so that inner healing can take place, and we can use the pink ray in Verbena to comfort and support us during this time.

Level of healing	Aromatherapy	Colour therapy
Physical	Detoxifies the liver	green to liver
	relieves cramps, indigestion, flatulence	green to stomach
	stimulates digestion and action of the bile	green to stomach
	softens skin and reduces puffiness	green to whole body
Emotional	use for shock, stress, grief, hurt by calming underlying tension	green to whole body, inhalation, colour breathing
	promotes loving relationships and sexual satisfaction through sharing and self-love	green to heart chakra
Mental	fights depression, acting as a tonic for the mind	pink to crown chakra
	relaxes and calms lower mind	green to back of the head
	helps the mind tune in to the heart	green to the crown chakra
Spiritual	breathes new life into us, brings new beginnings	green to the crown chakra
	creates space to grow spiritually	green to the whole aura

Precautions: Possible sensitisation due to photo-toxicity in some cases.

Affirmations: With the green ray of Verbena I am in harmony and balance.

VETIVERT

ANDROPOGON MURICATUS/VETIVERIA ZIZANOIDES
Healing colours/s: yellow
Colour aroma treatment/s: colour massage, colour aroma bath, perfume,
colour aroma lamps and diffusers, colour breathing, aromatic candles
Chakra affinity: solar-plexus
Life qualities: Decisiveness with flexibility, centredness, wisdom

Colour signature: Vetivert is a tall, tufted perennial scented grass with a
straight stem, which is coloured a rich golden-yellow. The roots from which
the dark amber oil is made has a fine fragrance. The strong golden colour
signature and straightness of the plant itself makes an excellent aid for
centring in order to find the core of one's own being and helping forge the
mind-body connection. Since the solar-plexus has a sympathetic frequency to the colour yellow, this oil works through this chakra to expand
one's personal power and self-confidence. Like most yellow oils, Vetivert
is good for skin care and for cleansing the blood stream of toxins. Its connection to the nervous system makes it very relaxing and valuable in baths
and massages especially if you are suffering from nervous exhaustion.

Level of healing	Aromatherapy	Colour therapy
Physical	arthritis, muscular aches and pains, sprains, stiffness, rheumatism	yellow over lower body
	acne and oily skin	yellow irradiation
	cuts and wounds	yellow to affected area
	increases blood flow and oxygen supply to the system	yellow to the soles of the feet
	tonic to the reproductive system	yellow to the pelvis
Emotional	treatment of stress and emotional weakness	yellow over solar-plexus
	calming and grounding	yellow to solar-plexus
	feeling disconnected, emotional burn-out	yellow to solar-plexus
	dispelling fear and anxiety	yellow to solar-plexus

Mental	brings peace and tranquility to the mind, use for insomnia, depression, debility	yellow to solar-plexus
	nervous tension	yellow to soles of feet
	disorientation	yellow to solar-plexus
Spiritual	shield of protection to the aura spiritual calmness by feeling grounded finding purpose in life	gold colour breathing gold gemstone to base chakra meditation using gold

Precautions: None that are apparent.

Affirmations: With Vetivert I feel calmly centred and know what action I must take.

VIOLET

Viola odorata

Healing colours/s: violet and green
Colour aroma treatment/s: colour compresses, colour aroma bath, colour nutrition, colour aroma meditation, perfume, colour reflexology
Chakra affinity: crown and heart
Life qualities: Peace, faith, service, piety, spirituality, mysticism

Colour signature: The oil is made from the fresh flowers of this small perennial plant. The oil vibrates on the violet ray but also contains green energy from the dark green heart-shaped leaves which helps promote the flow of energy between the heart and crown chakras. This opening of the heart and spirit allows love and friendship to flow. Violet is the colour of spirituality and service and the cleansing and transforming qualities are reflected in the fragile violet flowers. The affinity with the vibrations in the crown chakra make violet a healing colour for the brain, allowing

226

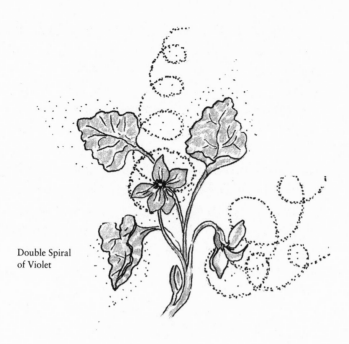

Double Spiral
of Violet

energy to come through from the higher mind. Violet flowers are antiseptic and have been reported to have pain-killing properties, and this is because they have a soporific effect on the conscious mind. Violet flowers were considered a good remedy against evil spirits, and the oil can be used for personal protection against harmful influences. On a physical level violet acts as a tonic to the kidneys, the seat of life force energy, and is able to disperse blocked energy in all the chakras, from the base to the crown.

Level of healing	Aromatherapy	Colour therapy
Physical	cleansing kidneys and congestion in lower body	violet over kidneys
	liver decongestant	violet over liver
	breathing and respiratory tract problems	violet over chest and throat
	soothes inflammation, pain-killing properties ease rheumatism, gout, fibrosis	violet over affected area

227

Emotional	restores libido especially during menopause	violet over base and sacral chakra
	balances emotions	violet over pituitary gland
	comforts and strengthens the heart	violet over the heart chakra
Mental	relieves congestion in head	violet over crown
	headaches, fits, giddiness	violet over crown
	insomnia, nervous exhaustion	violet over crown
Spiritual	helps search for truth and beauty	violet colour breathing
	bringer of faith and communion the spirit	meditation using violet

Precautions: None known

Affirmations: Through the Violet ray I appreciate the beauty in all things. With the colour violet I show my gratitude through service to others.

YARROW

Achillea millefolium
Healing colours/s: indigo
Colour aroma treatment/s: colour breathing, colour aroma lamps, colour inhaler, room spray mists, skin care lotions and perfumes.
Chakra affinity: third eye
Life qualities: insight, vision, integrity, thoughtfulness, intuition, composure

Colour signature: This common bush is often found in hedgerows and has fern-like feathery leaves with pink and white flowers. Yarrow essential oil is spicy but sweet, and its dark blue colouring reveals its true colour signature, which includes a small amount of red energy. Since ancient times, Yarrow has been considered a sacred herb and used for divination and to ward off evil spirits in homes and churches. The Indigo frequency opens the third eye chakra, and this is probably why in Scotland young maidens

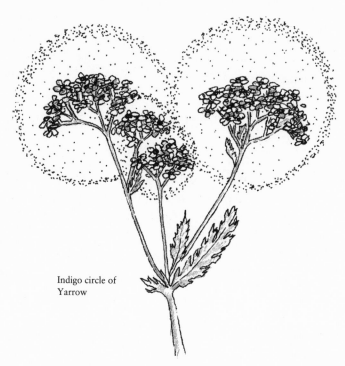

Indigo circle of
Yarrow

placed a sprig of Yarrow under their pillows in order to dream of true
love. Like all deep blue oils, Yarrow is cooling and reduces high body temperature. It has been also been used for hundreds of years as a wound healer
as it has an all healing action, reducing inflammation. It is best used for
the treatment of such problems as colds, diabetes and cancer. Indigo has
the vibration which penetrates the bone marrow, cleansing and healing
the cells at cellular level.

Level of healing	Aromatherapy	Colour therapy
Physical	cooling and promotes healing to cuts, burns, wounds, varicose veins, tones the skin, acne, eczema	indigo to affected area
	lowers blood pressure, rheumatoid arthritis, thrombosis,	indigo to feet, legs, joints
	indigestion, cramp, flatulence, haemorrhoids, constipation	indigo to stomach, liver
	colds, fevers, flu	indigo to chest in acute cases

Emotional	dissipates grief, loss, rejection, through inner calmness and balance	indigo to third eye chakra and throat
Mental	hypertension, insomnia, stress related conditions	Indigo to third eye
Spiritual	Opens the third eye to inner vision so helps self-development through dreams	Indigo to third eye

Precautions: Avoid during pregnancy, non-toxic, generally non-irritant.

Affirmations: Indigo energy cleanses my cells of impurities and releases my pain. With the Indigo ray in Yarrow I am totally protected from harmful vibrations.

YLANG YLANG

CANANGA ODORATA

Healing colours/s: pink, magenta, (yellow)
Colour aroma treatment/s: colour bath, colour massage, perfume, colour room diffuser, colour aroma lamps, colour candles, spray mists
Chakra affinity: base and heart
Life qualities: unifying, sensual, self-confident, uplifted, relaxed, awakened

Colour signature: Ylang Ylang is a very unusual oil derived from a tall tropical tree with large tender fragrant flowers which can be pink, mauve or yellow. The beautiful yellow flowers are considered best for essential oil, which has a powerful intoxicating aroma. Ylang Ylang has a frequency which resonates with our emotional or astral body, and is particularly useful in healing at this level. If the oil is made from yellow flowers it will have a strong effect on the nervous system which has a euphoric action and making it good for treatment of stress. The pink ray in Ylang Ylang works on the heart and also slows breathing allowing us to relax and to develop our sensitivity to other people's feelings. The red content in the pink frequency of Ylang Ylang, helps with sexual disorders of emotional origin. The warming and unifying energy of Ylang Ylang helps us know ourselves better and this awareness brings with it joy and contentment, as we understand who we are and why we are here.

Level of healing	Aromatherapy	Colour therapy
Physical	relaxes muscles, relieving heart palpitations, reduces high blood pressure, hyperventilation	pink/green light therapy over the heart
	promotes hair growth and a healthy skin	pink to whole body, soles of feet
Emotional	soothes and inhibits anger and frustration	pink light therapy to heart and foot reflex
	reaching out to others and sharing of self without losing personal power	magenta to solar-plexus
	developing self-love and being in touch with your body	pink to sacral chakra
Mental	anti-depressant, as it is a euphoric it is good for mental stress	magenta light on the base, green on the head to polarise energy.
Spiritual	Helps you live in the present without expectations	red over base chakra
	contentment through love and acceptance of who you are	magenta to whole aura

Precautions: Use in moderation. Like the colour yellow, too much Ylang Ylang can lead to headaches and nausea.

Affirmations: With the pink ray, my life is relaxed and I draw abundance to me. (Place a drop of oil directly on the pulse before saying the affirmation)

231

BIBLIOGRAPHY

The Directory of Essential Oils	Wanda Sellar	The C.W. Daniel Company
Subtle Aromatherapy	Patricia Davis	The C.W. Daniel Company
The Fragrant Mind	Valerie Ann Worwood	Doubleday Books – UK
Colour	Rudolph Steiner	Rudolph Steiner Press
The Rainbow Masters	'Dharma'	American West Distributors
Colour Psychology and Colour Therapy	Faber Birren	Citadel Press
Illustrated Encyclopaedia of Essential Oils	Julia Lawless	Element Books
The Art of Aromatherapy	Robert Tisserand	The C.W. Daniel Company
The Magna Book of Roses	Jo Finnis	Magna Books
Frontiers of Health	Christine Page	The C.W. Daniel Company

Index

Note: Page references in **bold** type refer to the main entries for essentials oils.